THE CONQUEST OF DEAFNESS

The Conquest of Deafness

A History of the Long Struggle to
Make Possible Normal Living to Those
Handicapped by Lack of Normal Hearing

RUTH E. BENDER, PH.D.

*Former Associate Clinical Professor,
Case Western Reserve
University, and Former Principal,
Preschool Hearing Program,
Cleveland Hearing and Speech Center*

The Interstate Printers & Publishers, Inc.
Danville, Illinois

Library of Congress Catalog Card No. 81-85399

ISBN 0-8134-2227-2

To David

Contents

LIST OF ILLUSTRATIONS

(grouped on pages 87 through 94)

ACKNOWLEDGMENTS

In a work of this scope it would be impracticable to give individual acknowledgment to all those who, either through professional position or personal interest, gave invaluable assistance to the writer. To all these people the writer wishes to extend sincere thanks for their patience and support.

Particular appreciation and acknowledgment must go to the personnel of the libraries of Western Reserve University, the Cleveland Public Library, the Armed Forces Library, in Cleveland, Ohio, The Volta Bureau and the library of Gallaudet College in Washington, D.C., as well as the New York Public Library and the Library of Congress.

Genuine gratitude is due Dr. Richard M. Flower for his sincere interest and professional guidance, and we must acknowledge special assistance and warmhearted co-operation from Dr. Tyson and Dr. Wright of Manchester University, England, Annetta Aarsen of Lisse and Dr. Groen of Groningen, Netherlands, and Dr. Maesse of Hamburg, Germany.

Foreword to The Third Edition

Dr. Ruth Bender's book *Conquest of Deafness* was first published in 1960, and a chapter was added for a second edition which appeared in 1970. Because of the scholarship which is evident throughout the book, it immediately became an authoritative work on historical developments pertaining to deaf people and in particular to their education. Many of the references (in other works) to the history of education of the deaf are based on Dr. Bender's original research.

This third edition was prompted by four events. First, two professors of the National Technical Institute for the Deaf at Rochester Institute of Technology, Ed Scouten and Ross Stuckless, brought to my attention the fact that this classic was no longer in print and that there were no plans for its reprinting. They were asked to pursue the matter and did so.

Second, 1981 marks the International Year of Disabled Persons, and it is fitting that the book be reintroduced as part of the observance of a year of special significance to handicapped persons around the world.

Third, Dr. Bender, now retired and living in Indiana, visited NTID at RIT and graciously assigned the copyright to our care.

Fourth, the events of the 1960's and 1970's have produced unprecedented change in the lives of hearing-impaired children and adults, and it was our feeling that these events should be brought together as an update of Dr. Bender's first edition. No educator of the deaf has been more active in these events at the national level than Dr. S. Richard Silverman. When he agreed to add a 1960-1980 update to Dr. Bender's book, the pieces fell into place.

It should be pointed out that the text of the first nine chapters is unchanged from that of Dr. Bender's first edition. Only Dr. Silverman's concluding chapter is added and references in this chapter are presented as an appendix to Dr. Bender's original bibliography.

We also draw the reader's attention to Dr. Bender's concluding chapter of her second edition, in which she discusses events of the 1960's. That chapter is not included in this third edition because we wanted to step back and look at the general tone of the full past two decades. If the reader is in possession of the second edition, value it.

If I were asked to name the four or five most important books concerning the education of hearing-impaired children, *Conquest of Deafness* would certainly be among them. It is a privilege for NTID at RIT to have a part in assuring that this significant work remains available to professionals, to parents, and to deaf people themselves.

William E. Castle
Vice President, RIT
and Director, NTID

INTRODUCTION

Hearing loss, as an affliction of mankind, has apparently been with us for as long as man himself. It has been, and still is, called by a variety of names. "Deafness" is the most universal, and also probably the most misunderstood of these titles. It seems to imply a total inability to hear. This is seldom the case.

In 1938, a definition of the terms for hearing loss was formulated by a special committee on nomenclature, for the Conference of Executives of American Schools for the Deaf. This is their statement:

> Finally, these definitions are proposed:
> 1. The Deaf: Those in whom the sense of hearing is non-functional for the ordinary purpose of life. This general group is made up of two distinct classes based entirely on the time of loss of hearing.
>   a. The congenitally deaf—those who are born deaf.
>   b. The adventitiously deaf—those who are born with normal hearing but in whom the sense of hearing became non-functional later through illness or accident.
> 2. The Hard-of-Hearing: Those in whom the sense of hearing, although defective, is functional, with or without a hearing aid. (203)

Hardy contrasts the terms in reference to the educational approach necessary for the child with impaired hearing. The hard-of-hearing child is one who has enough auditory discrimination to acquire some usable degree of oral language through hearing, but needs training in both visual and auditory patterns for complete language acquisition. The deaf child must acquire his language largely through visual patterns (67) with what additional clues are possible by means of residual hearing. (63).

Because lack of hearing has always been accompanied by lack of speech, hearing being the normal route by which we learn to speak, the words "dumb" and "mute" have always had a close association with the word "deaf." Even today, in spite of the prevalence of oral speech among the deaf, they are still referred to as "deaf and dumb" and "deaf-mute" in most countries and most languages.

This account of the history of the deaf and their education will, of necessity, use the terms applied to them in the writings that have come down to us through the years. We are not dealing, however, with people who are truly mute, but with those who are deaf and consequently had not learned to speak. The terms "deaf and dumb" and "deaf-mute" are used in this treatise merely because they were the words historically used, and not as accurate descriptions of the condition of the persons designated.

Evidence of arthritis is clearly revealed in the bones of prehistoric animals. (143) No such evidence is possible to prove the earliest presence of deafness. We must wait for man's written records. But as these records come into existence, we find deafness recorded as a long-familiar and all-too-frequent occurrence.

The first historians were content merely to comment on lack of hearing, and more particularly, lack of speech in some of their contemporaries. As philosophy and medical science advanced, this curious double phenomenon attracted more and more attention and comment. In each succeeding era, the twin afflictions of hearing loss and lack of language were described and interpreted according to the medical and educational outlook of that day. When ignorance, superstition, and neglect were the lot of the handicapped, the deaf had their full measure of suffering. As education and scientific knowledge progressed, and the condition of the common people improved, the deaf were included in the general benefits. Not infrequently, their particular problems secured for them the attention of philosophers and educators in advance of general educational progress.

One purpose of this work is to trace this development in the understanding of deafness and education of the deaf. In order to have a valid understanding of the position of the deaf at any time, it is important to see them always within the educational and social structure of that time. Accordingly, in this work, a brief survey of the times and circumstances surrounding each epoch will precede a description of that period in the education of the deaf.

By reason of their brevity, many of the allusions to general education in various periods may appear somewhat naive in their over-simplification. Probably most of the events in the education of the deaf were results of local circumstances. Nevertheless, there was some reflection of the general patterns of the day in the handling of the deaf, so that these comments have a valid function and are, therefore, included.

To make the bibliographical source material as practically useful as possible, a double system of notes has been arranged.

The superior letters [a] refer to notes immediately available at the bottom of the page.

The bibliographical references in the first nine chapters are indicated by numbers, thus: (73) will lead the reader to *Hill, Moritz* in the bibliography. But the bibliography has been arranged alphabetically by authors, and if more than one work by the same author is cited, as in the case of Hill, the reference is (73,b), which indicates Hill's *Elementar-Lese-und Sprachbuch*. Page references are in many cases added, to facilitate easy reference.

References cited in chapter 10, "1960-1980 in the U.S." are by author and year of publication, and these follow the bibliography for the first nine chapters.

THE CONQUEST OF DEAFNESS

Chapter 1

In Early Times

In the early history of mankind, the family was the basic unit of society. Children observed their elders as they went about their tasks of daily living. As children do in all times, they imitated these activities in spontaneous play, father in the games of hunting, mother in her preparation of food and clothing.

As early as they were able, the children took part with their elders in the ever-present struggle for existence. As their games turned to earnest work, their small hands contributed to the family a share of the basic necessities for living. (49)

From earliest times, families were banded together into tribes for mutual help and protection. Traditional rites and customs evolved, to hold the tribe together, and guide their activities according to the experience of the past. With no written language, tribal lore was preserved and handed on by means of story-telling, pantomimic dances, and dramatic presentations.

At puberty, the young people were initiated into full membership in the tribe by traditional rites and ceremonies. Weeks of intensive preparation in a secluded spot often preceded the final graduation exercises. Thus much of the tradition of the past was handed down to the next generation. After these initiations, the young people assumed full responsibility for citizenship, to pass on, in their turn, the wisdom of the past.

In such a system of education, no special provision needed to be made for the handicapped, if they survived the rigors of primitive life. In many cases, they did not survive. It is known that among many primitive people, those who could not contribute their share to the needs of the tribe, were not allowed to live. Infants who appeared to be deformed or weak were often destroyed at birth.

Since hearing loss is not a visible handicap at an early age, nor in its early stages, it is not known how these unfortunates were regarded by their families and associates. But it is unlikely that the efforts made for their protection in more advanced stages of society could have been common in earlier times.

As civilization became more complex and the organization of society more intricate, laws were drawn up in greater detail to carry out the current interpretation of justice in men's dealings with one another. In the code of Hammurabi (2067-2025 B.C.) (49), specific provision was made for the punishment of various misdemeanors. The penalties imposed were often in the form of symbolic retaliation. The tongue that spoke perjury was cut out; the eye that looked on forbidden secrets was destroyed; the hand that struck a father was cut off. Even the surgeon whose lack of skill cost his patient the loss of life or limb paid for his mistake by the loss of his own hand. (116; 147,a)

It is in the early body of Hebrew law that we find the first known provision for the protection of the deaf.

The Hebrew people of early times stood out from their neighbors in several ways: in their concept of God as a personal deity, who concerns Himself with justice and mercy in the lives of His people; in their acceptance of personal responsibility for high moral and ethical standards; in the dignity of their womanhood; in their concern for the education of their children.

During their exile in Babylon (566 B.C.), the influences of the conflicting cultures and religions threatened the integrity and continuity of their own treasured traditions. To counteract such influences, the elders and priests augmented the traditional teaching of Hebrew children in the home by establishing elementary classes in the synagogue, or in a room adjoining the synagogue. (49)

It was consistent, therefore, for the Hebrew people to look with compassion upon the unfortunate members of their society and to provide for their welfare. They believed firmly that such afflicted ones came from the hand of the Lord and were under His special protection.

And the Lord said unto him, Who hath made man's mouth? Or who maketh the dumb or deaf, or the seeing or the blind? Have not I, the Lord?[a]

Thou shalt not curse the deaf nor put a stumbling block before the blind, but shalt fear thy God.[b]

This same compassion for the unfortunate was later expressed by Christ.

The Hebrew laws, in general, classed the deaf and dumb with the mentally defective and with children in assuming that they were not able to take normal adult responsibility.

If one exposes his cattle to the sun, or he places them in the custody of a deaf-mute, a fool, or a minor, and they break away and do damage, he is liable. (96: Chap. IV, Mishna I, p. 131, Baba Kamma, 6:2 and 4, p. 339)

The deaf-mute was not considered competent as a witness to any transaction, for all testimony was given orally. A deaf-mute could not be punished if he or his ox injured someone, but injury to him or his possessions was punishable. The man who was a deaf-mute, and the man who was only deaf but had speech, were allowed to transact business with movable goods, but could not possess real estate. The man who was only dumb, but could hear and understand language, was placed under no legal restrictions. He could transact any manner of business, and was held responsible for his own actions and property.

Since the deaf-mute had no legal power of acquiring property, if he found anything he was not entitled to, it could be taken away from him. The Rabbis, however, considered this robbery, and, in order to preserve the peace of the community, they decided that such property must be returned to the finder.

According to Biblical law, marriage of deaf-mutes was not valid, but the Rabbis sanctioned such marriage when contracted by signs. (162).

The Greeks on their peninsula in the Mediterranean, developed a culture and a philosophy of education to which our present civilization is still indebted. The education of their children was strictly supervised, from early childhood, to insure a full, rounded development of body, mind, and spirit. The fathers of Greek families and the elders of the State took deep pride in guiding the development of their sons in every detail.

[a]Exodus 4:11. Holy Bible (King James Version)
[b]Leviticus 19:14. Holy Bible (King James Version)

But they were interested mainly in the education of their sons, not their daughters. Also, these were only the sons of the ruling class, who formed a very small fraction of the population. The wealth and leisure which made it possible for these men to develop Greek culture rested heavily on the backs of thousands of toiling slaves. For these there was no education, only hard physical labor. Here and there a master might free a favorite slave who showed exceptional promise, and grant him some of the advantages of the privileged class. But the general masses of the people had no such advantages.

Even the sons of the wealthy were favored only if they gave promise of individual fitness. In both Sparta and Athens, infants were examined at birth by elders of the State, before they were acknowledged by the family. If they showed signs of imperfection, they were exposed on a mountainside to die.

Knowledge of cause and effect in the functions of the human mind and body was very meager in those days. Language and speech were considered to be instinctive rather than acquired. So it appeared ridiculous to try to teach language where is did not exist naturally.

Aristotle (355 B.C.) discussed the phenomenon in his "History of Animals," in these words:

> Viviparous quadrupeds utter vocal sounds of different kinds, but they have no power of converse. In fact, this power, or language, is peculiar to man. For while the capability of talking implies the capability of uttering sounds, the converse does not hold good. Men that are deaf are in all cases also dumb; that is, they can make vocal sounds, but they cannot speak. Children, just as they have no control over other parts, so have no control, at first, over the tongue; but it is so far imperfect, and only frees and detaches itself by degrees, so that in the interval children for the most part lisp and stutter. (7,a: Book IV, No. 9)

The sentence on deafness was lifted out of its context by later writers and quoted as final authority on the deaf.

It may be translated literally in this fashion:

> Those who become deaf from birth also become altogether speechless. Voice is certainly not lacking, but there is no speech. (7,b)

Unfortunately, the words *"kophoi"* meaning "deaf," and *"eneos"* meaning "speechless," had also taken on the meanings "dumb" and "stupid" in some instances. Isolated from its accompanying paragraph, the translation of the sentence became so distorted that it was quoted by some writers, to say,

Those who are born deaf all become senseless and incapable of reason. (75)

This pronouncement was especially disastrous to the deaf, since the writings of Aristotle were accepted without question for hundreds of years, down through the Middle Ages. No one was even curious to explore the possible capabilities of the deaf, since the word of authority on their incapability had already been pronounced.

Hippocrates of Cos (460 B.C.) (75, p. 63) the great physician, developed some knowledge of the nature of infections in the middle ear. He also commented on the lack of speech in those deaf from birth as evidence that speech, to be intelligible, depends upon a proper action of the tongue. (8,b) A comprehension of the relationship between hearing and speech seemed to be vague, to say the least, for Hippocrates, and for medical men for centuries after him.

It is evident that the deaf and dumb have always communicated to some extent by pantomimic signs and gestures. Socrates (386 B.C.) (38) commented on this fact in his discussion with Hermogenes and Cratylus concerning the names of things:

SOCRATES—
But answer me this question: If we had neither voice nor tongue, and yet wished to manifest things to one another, should we not, like those which are at present mute, endeavor to signify our meaning by the hands, head, and other parts of the body?
HERMOGENES—
How could it be otherwise, Socrates?
SOCRATES—
I think, therefore, that if we wished to signify that which is upwards and light, we should raise our hands toward the heavens, imitating the nature of the thing itself; but that if we wished to indicate things downwards and heavy, we should point with our hands to the earth. And again, if we were desirous of signifying a running horse, or any other animal, you know, that we would fashion the gestures and figures of our bodies, as near as possible, to a similitude of those things.
HERMOGENES—
How could it be otherwise, Socrates? (106, pp. 94-95)

With the conquest of Greece by Rome, much of Greek culture and thought was transplanted to the West. The Romans were fascinated by the superior education of the conquered Greeks, and set out to appropriate it for their sons. They also adapted it to conform more closely to their ways of thinking. The practical and legal aspects were emphasized, while the softer, more artistic elements were made secondary.

Roman society, too, had a privileged class of citizens and free men, and a vast population of slaves. The latter were seldom considered in the learned debates in the Roman Senate concerning the rights of men.

Roman infants who did not meet the accepted standards of physical perfection were laid at the base of the statues in the public square to be torn to pieces by dogs. It has been suggested by some writers that deaf babies were included in this exposure. But this is hardly probable, since any hearing loss would not have been evident at so early an age.

It has been said that Romulus, the legendary founder of Rome, forbade the destruction of children under the age of three unless they showed gross deformity at birth. Those who later appeared likely to become a liability to the State were allowed to be murdered at three years of age. This, according to Dionysius of Halicarnassus, was early Roman practice. (38; 46)

One individual case of educational opportunity offered a deaf child is recorded by Pliny, the Elder, in his Natural History (77 A.D.). (147,e) Quintus Pedius was the deaf and dumb son of Quintus Pedius, the Consul, and co-heir with Caesar Augustus. Apparently, Augustus took an interest in his colleague's afflicted son, and approved painting lessons for the boy, who, it was said, became very proficient in the art.

There is no record that this accomplishment had any influence on the fate of others with similar handicaps. Pliny, in the same book, made the comment that

> When one is first of all denied hearing, he is also robbed of the power of talking, and there are no persons born deaf who are not also dumb. (75)

Claudius Galen, the eminent physician, compiled an encyclopedia of the medical knowledge of his time (170 A.D.). (147,b,d) He assumed a common origin in the brain for speech and hearing, and presented the corollary that an injury in this area would result, automatically, in both deafness and dumbness. The existence of a functional relationship between the two did not seem to have occurred to him nor to his contemporaries.

The ancient Roman law placed the deaf and dumb in the category of those who had no intelligence and therefore no legal rights. Some concession was made for those who were only deaf or only dumb.

In the code of laws compiled by the Emperor Justinian, (530 A.D.), the classification and legal rights of the deaf and dumb were stated in this fashion:

1. The deaf and dumb in whom both infirmities were present from birth: these were without legal rights or obligations. Guardians appointed for them by law were to have complete charge of their affairs.

2. Those who became deaf and dumb from causes arising after birth: if these people had acquired a knowledge of letters before their affliction, they were allowed to conduct their own affairs by means of writing. This included marriage contracts, which were denied the previous class.

3. Those deaf from birth, but not dumb, and

4. Those deaf from causes arising after birth, but not dumb: these two classes were assumed to have the use of language to a sufficient degree to carry on the responsibilities of their own lives. No restrictions seem to have been placed on their legal rights. (They would undoubtedly be classified today as the hard of hearing and deafened.)

5. Those who were dumb only, either from birth or from later causes: this classification is obscure. No restrictions were placed on these people, since it was assumed they could understand spoken language and reply in writing. (8,a; 37; 114; 147,c)

The law expressly stated that no discrimination was to be made between men and women in the administration of these rules.

From the dawn of history into the early Christian era, there was little place in society for the handicapped. Since their presence in the group was often an economic calamity, they were either destroyed or allowed to shift for themselves, without group support or consideration. Medical knowledge about hearing and speech was scanty and inaccurate and gave little help toward the understanding of the problems of the deaf.

Chapter 2

The Period of the Rise and Spread of Christianity

(30-1400 A.D.)

Roman imperialism held within its own character the forces of its own destruction. It exploited what it conquered, sapping the vitality of the invaded territories for its own fattening. In the end, all wealth and power were gathered into the hands of so few that the whole structure of Roman society became top-heavy. The stabilizing balance of a middle class virtually disappeared. The impoverished and hungry peasantry had neither will nor strength to oppose either their own rulers or their enemies from the outside.

When, in the fourth and fifth centuries after Christ, the barbarians from the North pushed against the Roman lines, there was little to resist them. The integrity and unity of the Roman empire vanished. Anarchy and dissension took its place. Centuries were to pass before a body of responsible rulers could again be established. (49)

Through this changing world walked the early Christians, with their strange new doctrine of the brotherhood of all men.

The pagan religions of those times were unethical and immoral to an extreme that is difficult for us to realize today. Against this background, the teachings of Jesus stood out in bright, warm contrast.

24

He was concerned about the plight of the handicapped and frequently remedied their situation with miraculous cures. Watching him, his followers developed a degree of compassion that was strange to their neighbors, and led to the growth of more humanistic attitudes in society.

> Now when John (the Baptist) heard in prison about the deeds of the Christ, he sent word by his disciples and said to him, "Are you he who is to come or shall we look for another?" And Jesus answered them, "Go and tell him (John) what you hear and see: the blind receive their sight and the lame walk, lepers are cleansed and the deaf hear, and the dead are raised up, and the poor have good news preached to them. And blessed is he who takes no offense at me." [a,b]
> And they were astonished beyond measure, saying, "He has done all things well; he even makes the deaf hear and the dumb speak."[c]

The development of a new philosophy and a new religion was not accepted easily. Driven by persecution into secrecy and isolation, the early Christians, in many places, banded together in communal living, under the leadership of holy men. From these communities, religious groups were eventually organized under definite rules of living, which developed into monastic orders. (49)

For the common people, life was still a bitter struggle for the bare essentials of living. The greater part of the meager production of their labor was taken in rent and taxes. They were swept by recurring plagues and diseases, which were attributed to supernatural causes. Whether these were caused by the malicious agency of hostile spirits or were instruments of Divine punishment made little difference. Ill-fed and ignorant of the most elementary rules of health and sanitation, the people were an easy prey to these catastrophes. In their misery, their only help came from the long-robed men and women of the religious orders, who ventured out of the doors of their monasteries for little else but such errands of mercy.

The monasteries became the guardians of the literature of the past. Long hours were spent in copying manuscripts of ancient writers, both to preserve them and to share them with other monasteries.

Of these ancient writers, one of the most highly revered was Aristotle. Another was St. Augustine, a church father in the beginning of the fourth century, A. D. He emphasized the doctrine of un-

[a] Matthew 11:2-6. Holy Bible, Revised Standard Version
[b] Luke 7:18-22. Holy Bible, Revised Standard Version
[c] Mark 7:37. Holy Bible, Revised Standard Version

questioning faith as opposed to dependence on sense and reason.
(49) As one proof of the natural depravity of man, with the sins of
the fathers visited on the children, he pointed out babies who were
handicapped from birth.

The passage referred to may be freely translated thus:

> We acknowledge, indeed, how much pertains to our own trans-
> gressions: from what source of culpability does it come that innocent
> ones deserve to be born sometimes blind, sometimes deaf, which
> defect, indeed, hinders faith itself, by the witness of the Apostle, who
> says, "Faith comes by hearing. (Rom. X, 17)." Now, truly, what bears
> out the assertion that the soul of the "innocent" is in the image of God,
> inasmuch as the liberation of the one born foolish is by his rich gift, if
> not that the bad merited by the parents is transmitted to the children?
> (11)

There was little room in the philosphy of these times for exploring the possibilities of medical and educational progress, especially
in the area of the handicapped. But they were included in the many
accounts of miraculous visitations with which the literature is filled.

In the northern section of the island that is now Britain,
Ceowulph (673-735), king of Northumbria, took a great interest in
encouraging the advance of things spiritual and educational. Among
other efforts along these lines, he commissioned the Venerable
Bede, priest of the abbey of Jarrow (17), to write a history of the
church and of the Anglo-Saxon people.

The Venerable Bede was most thorough and detailed in carrying
out his commission. His book is crowded with devils, spirits, and
miracles. The miracles described were largely miracles of healing,
performed by godly priests and bishops, sometimes by the
bestowal of their blessing, sometimes by the unwitting touch of
their garments or possessions.

According to Bede's account, there lived, about 685, a bishop of
Hagulstad, who was later called St. John of Beverly. He had a
building, sheltered in a wood not far from his church, that he was
accustomed to use as a retreat. It was his practice to retire to this
secluded spot, with a number of his co-workers and helpers, on
various religious occasions.

The Venerable Bede described one such occasion:

> Being come thither once at the beginning of Lent, to stay, he com-
> manded his followers to find out some poor person labouring under
> any grievous infirmity, or want, whom he might keep with him during
> those days, by way of alms, for so he was always used to do.
> There was in a village not far off, a certain dumb youth, known to

the bishop, for he often used to come into his presence to receive alms, and had never been able to speak one word. Besides, he had so much scurf and scabs on his head that no hair ever grew on the top of it, but only some scattered hairs in a circle round about. The bishop caused this young man to be brought, and a little cottage to be made for him within the enclosure of the dwelling, in which he might reside, and receive a daily allowance from him. When one week of Lent was over, the next Sunday he caused the poor man to come in to him, and ordered him to put his tongue out of his mouth and show it to him; then laying hold of his chin, he made the sign of the cross on his tongue, directing him to draw it back into his mouth and to speak. "Pronounce some word," said he, "say yea." . . . The youth's tongue was immediately loosed, and he said what he was ordered. The bishop then pronouncing the names of the letters, directed him to say A; he did so and afterward B, which he also did. When he had named all the letters after the bishop, the latter proceeded to put syllables and words to him, which being also repeated by him, he commanded him to utter whole sentences, and he did it. Nor did he cease, all that day and the next night, as long as he could keep awake, as those who were present, relate, to talk something and to express his private thoughts and will to others, which he could never do before. . . . The bishop, rejoicing at his recovery of speech, ordered the physician to take in hand the cure of his scurfed head. He did so, and with the help of the bishop's blessing and prayers, a good head of hair grew as the flesh was healed. (17)

This has been, perhaps, the most frequently quoted incident from the literature of the Middle Ages concerning the recovery of speech. Although no mention was made of deafness, the most usual interpretation of the story called the man a deaf-mute, and St. John of Beverly the first teacher of the deaf. (8,a; 20; 118; 124)

It has also been interpreted as a description of recovery from aphasia. (75)

The story, as it stands, hardly supports either interpretation. Most authorities suggest that the young man's period of teaching no doubt covered a much longer period of time than the one week recorded by Bede.

With the growth of Christianity, there began to develop a more humane interest in the lot of the common man. But such few glimpses as we have of the deaf during these times are completely imbedded in the stories of miraculous healing and instantaneous recoveries from lifelong afflictions. There is no description of any actual attempt at teaching the deaf. Probably there were no such attempts.

Chapter 3

The Re-Awakening

(1400-1500)

Many things contributed to the re-awakening and re-development of science, education, and culture, which began in the fourteenth century. Once more a class possessing wealth and leisure grew up, cradled in the courts of southern France. (49) Artists, scholars, and poets were given shelter and patronage. Poetry and song were expressed in native languages, instead of in ancient Latin, and were used to celebrate the great events of the day. These stories were sung from court to court by traveling troubadour knights, and served to spread the knowledge.

Travel and discovery brought thrilling tales of strange lands, to fire men's imagination. The boundaries of geography were pushed back. Columbus discovered America, and, a quarter of a century later, Magellan sailed around the world. The earth was round, and the medieval geography books were in the discard. With them went many long-accepted ideas concerning science and medicine.

Perhaps the one single event that gave the greatest impetus to study was the invention of printing. The making of paper, developed from processes brought back by travelers to the Orient, was already an important industry in Europe by 1320. (38) Still the production of books was a slow, costly process and books were few and expensive.

About 1438, Johann Gutenberg, of Mainz, Germany, invented movable type and a practical process of printing. Rapidly, books were printed and distributed in amazing numbers. But the zeal for more learning out-paced the new process that made it available. (38)

The emphasis of study in the universities swung from the dusty scholasticism of the past to a fresh contemplation of humanity. (49)

Religious reforms re-emphasized individual responsibility for faith and salvation. Since the only road to such responsibility was by way of personal knowledge, education became a vital factor in the new Protestant churches.

The spread of learning encouraged the use of the common languages, for reading and writing as well as speaking. Another development was the inclusion of girls as well as boys in the scheme of education.

Among the learned men of the time who took notice of the deaf was Leonardo da Vinci. He made an interesting comment on lipreading as a comparison for the artist in depicting figures. The comment is taken from the passage Of the Parts of the Face, in his Precepts of the Painter, which is included in the Codice Atlantico, written sometime about 1499.

> A picture or any representation of figures ought to be done in such a way that those who see them may be able with ease to recognize from their attitudes what is passing through their minds. . . . Just so a deaf mute, who sees two people talking, although being himself deprived of the power of hearing, is none the less able to divine from the movements and gestures of the speakers the subject of their discussion.
>
> I once saw in Florence a man who had become deaf, who could not understand you if you spoke to him loudly, while if you spoke softly without letting the voice utter any sound he understood you merely from the movement of the lips. Perhaps, however, you will say to me: 'But does not a man who speaks loudly move his lips like one who speaks softly? And since one moves his lips like the other, will not he be understood like the other?' As to this, I leave the decision to the test of experience. Set someone to speak softly and then (louder), and watch the lips. C. A. 139 r.d. (90, p. 902)

Among the educational leaders of the new humanistic schools was one Roelof Huysman, born in Groningen, Netherlands, in 1443. During a period of study in Ferrara, Italy, he followed a usual custom among scholars, and Latinized his name to Rudolph Agricola. It was by this form that he was commonly known. He did much to spread the new humanistic education through Germany. (42, p. 304; 142)

One of his best-known books, written in Latin, *De Inventione Dialectica,* was published after his death. The dates of as many as eight editions of this book are given, ranging from 1521 to 1567. (189)

In this book he commented that:

> I have seen an individual, deaf from the cradle, and by consequence mute, who had learned to understand all that was written by other persons, and who expressed by writing all his thoughts, as if he had the use of words. (1)

This comment was taken up by a physician from the university of Padua, Italy, a man named Girolamo Cardano, commonly known as Jerome Cardan. He developed considerable knowledge of physiology, and was particularly concerned with the eyes, ears, mouth, and brain.

In his book called *Paralipomenon,* Third Book, Chapter Eight, there occurred this passage, titled "De Surdo et Muto literas edocto,"

> Concerning Deaf and Dumb taught letters Georgius Agricola refers, in his third book of *Inventione Dialectica* to having seen a man born deaf and dumb, who learned to read and write, so that he could express what he wished. Thus we can accomplish that a mute hear by reading and speak by writing. For by thinking his memory understands that *bread,* for example, means that thing which is eaten. He thus reads, by reason, even as in a picture; for by this means, although nothing is referred to voices, not only things, but actions and results are made known, and as from a picture the meaning of another picture is formed, so that by reasoning it may be understood, so also in letters. [a,b]

This was a revolutionary declaration. It broke down the long-established belief that the hearing of words was necessary for the understanding of ideas. It recognized the ability of the deaf to use reason.

[a] Refert Georgius Agricola in tertio suo libro de Inventione Dialectica vidisse hominem natum surdum et mutum, qui legere se scribere didicerit, sic ut significerat que vellet. Atque ita possumus officere ut mutus legendo audiet et scribendo loquatur. Nam ex cogitatione memoria comprehendit quod panis, gratia exempli, rem illam quae editur, significat. Legit itaque ratione velut in pictura; per eam enim licet ad voces non referatur, non solum res, sed actiones et successus declarantur. Et ut ex pictura visa picturam aliam effingere, sub ratione etiam significati licet; ita etiam in literia. (32,b)

[b] The title of the work is worth recording: Hieronymi Cardani, Mediolanensis Philosophi ac Medici Celeberrimi Operam, Tomas Decimus; *Quo Continentur Opuscula Miscellanea Ex Fragmentis et Paralipomenis,* (Lugduni: Sumptibus Joannis Antonii Huguetan et Marci Antonnii Ravaud, M·DC·LXIII (1663)

Jerome Cardan of Milan, Famous Philosopher and Physician; Ten Books, In which are contained A Little Miscellaneous Work from Fragments and Things Omitted.

Cardan, himself, was a brilliant but erratic scholar, with a background of instability and unhappiness. He was born in Paris, September 24, 1501, and handed over, according to a prevailing custom, to a nurse to bring up. She died of plague in his first month, and the baby had spots and carbuncles on his face. His mother took him back briefly but did not want him. He was taken into the home of Isidore del Reste, a friend of his father. Isidore obtained a new nurse, burned the baby's clothes, dipped him in vinegar, as a disinfectant, and handed him over, dripping wet.

He did not thrive in this home, either, and was transferred to another, where he lived until the age of three. Then he was taken back by his mother into her home in Milan, Italy. He was always in delicate health, and ill-treated in a family that was unstable and disturbed.

He studied medicine and received his degree as doctor of medicine at Padua, Italy, in 1526, and was married in 1531. He was extremely superstitious, and was rejected by the doctors in Milan. He was always poor, and troubled by the misdeeds of his two sons and the death of his daughter. His chief comfort was his grandson, Fazio, named for his father, whom he brought up from the age of three months.

He was a brilliant and prolific writer, producing many books on medicine and related subjects. He even elaborated a kind of code for teaching the deaf to read. But there is no evidence that he made any attempt to put it to practical use. (75, p. 80)

He died in Rome, September 20, 1576, at the age of 75. (42; 97)

From Spain came a fascinating story of a young man who reached fame and fortune in spite of the handicap of deafness.

Juan Fernandez Ximenes de Navarette was born in Logroño, Spain. The dates given for his birth range from October 3, 1526 to 1532. (12; 27; 40) At the age of three, an acute malady deprived him of his hearing, and consequently of his speech, so that he was commonly called El Mudo (The Mute). (27)

His parents placed him under the care of Fray Vicente de Santo Domingo, who instructed him in painting. He showed such early talent that his tutor suggested he should be sent to Italy to study painting. At fourteen, he went to Italy, where he remained for about twenty years. During this time he became an admirer and disciple of the great Titian at Venice, and imitated Titian in his own painting. (27; 61; 123)

Philip II of Spain was much interested in art, and extended his patronage and the support of his court to many artists. He was, at this time, in the process of decorating the walls of The Escorial. He hired one painter after another to decorate various sections of the edifice, and was frequently dissatisfied with the results, partly because the painters were not too talented, but also because he exerted considerable pressure on them for speed in completing their work. (11)

Luis Manrique, chief chaplain to the king, suggested his consideration of El Mudo's work. El Mudo submitted, as his part of the competition, a painting of the Baptism of Christ. The king accepted him, and El Mudo entered the service of Philip II of Spain in 1568.(12)

The young man justified his early promise. Many of his paintings became famous. Each seemed to have some particular quality which made it stand out as having special merit. The Burial of Lazarus used the effect of artificial light, with a man lighting a candle. In his scene of The Nativity, he arranged three sources of light, one shining from the Infant, one from the torch in Joseph's hand, and the third shed over the group of Shepherds. This picture is often called "Beautiful Shepherds," it is said, from the exclamation of his friend Tibaldi, upon seeing it.

In meeting the requirements of paintings requested for The Escorial, the painter worked under strict rules. His contract imposed on him the responsibility for furnishing his own colors and materials. He was forbidden to use any materials that would be unusual or difficult for another painter, following him, to acquire. The canvases were to be heavy and without seam. For this, they had to be especially woven. He was also responsible for the transportation of his paintings to The Escorial.

In painting figures, each standing figure was to be exactly 6¼ feet in height. If the figure of any particular saint was repeated, it was to be as if he painted a portrait, with the same features and same garments repeated, so that the saint might be readily identified. There was to be no cat nor dog nor other irreverent figure to distract the viewers from their worship. (12; 27)

But El Mudo had a sense of humor, and Philip II appears to have been indulgent. In his painting of The Holy Family, the heads are beautiful and expressive. But on one side of the group is a partridge and on the other side a dog and a cat engaged in a comical fight over a bone. (27)

In the cloister, at the head of The Escorial, El Mudo hung his painting of The Martyrdom of Saint James. He was then at enmity with Santayo, the king's secretary, and used his features as a model for the face of the executioner. Santayo begged to have it changed, but the king was too much a friend of El Mudo's to enter into the grudge.

Philip II seemed to have a special fondness for his deaf painter. The king often intervened to keep El Mudo from destroying those of his own works that he did not consider worthy, notably his picture of the Assumption, where the face of the Virgin was that of his own mother, who was very beautiful.

When Titian's celebrated painting of The Last Supper was ordered for the dining room of The Escorial, it proved, upon arrival, to be too long for the space it was to occupy. Philip II proposed to cut it down to the proper size. El Mudo begged to be allowed to copy it in smaller proportions, so that it could be used intact. Arguing with the king, by gestures and signs, he offered to complete the task in six months. But the king decided it was not worth the time and money involved, and had the picture cut to the required size. (27; 35, p. 283; 61)

A serious illness in 1571 sent El Mudo back to Logroño for a change of air, where he lived for three years on a pension from the king. Later he returned to Madrid and The Escorial and continued his work as painter for Philip II. Always in delicate health, he had finished only eight of the thirty-two paintings he had contracted to produce when he died in Toledo in 1579. [a] (12; 27; 98; 123)

Lope de Vega said of him:

> If heaven did not wish him to speak it was so that, according to my understanding, he should give more feeling to the subjects he painted. He gave them so much life with his unique brush that not being able to speak himself, he made them speak for him. (12, p. 107)

At about the same time when El Mudo was painting in Spain, there was in France another young man who, in spite of hearing loss, achieved fame in the field of literature. Pierre de Ronsard, born near Paris, September 11, 1524, was sent at the age of twelve to the court of François I, to be apprenticed as page to the Dauphin, the king's eldest son. The young prince, only eighteen, died three days after his new page's arrival at court. The boy was then attached to the service of another son of the king, and followed the fortunes of the royal family for years to come.

In August, 1540, while on a trip to Germany in attendance on a prince of the court of France, Ronsard was seized with severe attacks of fever, which continued after his return to Paris. These were accompanied by severe ear infections, which left him for a time totally deaf, then half-deaf for the rest of his life. (47)

---

[a] Gould stated that "he died in 1572, aged 40."

Although only sixteen at the time of this illness, Ronsard was already on the way to a brilliant career as soldier and diplomat. Realizing that his hearing loss would be a serious handicap in such a career, he immediately decided to "transfer the office of his ears to his eyes," and set himself to study by reading good books. His father, having no fortune to leave his son, had previously opposed his interest in such an unremunerative field as that of literature. He now withdrew his objections, only suggesting that Pierre study for a small clerical position, in order that he might have a living while he wrote.

Ronsard turned his brilliance and personality to his new career with the same fervor he had shown in the previous one. He became one of the best-known French poets of his time.

Nowhere, in all the large volume of his extant published poetry, did he seem to have time to bemoan his fate. His poems followed the romantic pattern of his day, extolling the beauties and virtues of people who caught his fancy, both historic and contemporary. (109)

His biographer made this comment about him:

> Truly, this young man of a mediocre family, but who knew how to make himself loved and respected by the most influential people, could have aspired to great fortune, being a courtier, diplomat, or following his father's example, a soldier. But would it not have been a loss to poetry, if a terrible illness had not suddenly forced him to renounce such careers? [a] (47,p. 4)

Another French poet, contemporary with Ronsard, Joachim Du Bellay (1522-1560), found resignation more difficult. According to his biographer, Du Bellay's hearing loss was partial but of long standing. His life was frequently interrupted by repeated ear infections. At one time, it was told, he was "confined to his room for a month by a troublesome deafness," so that he had not even the consolation of bidding farewell to Marguerite of France, the royal princess who took a special interest in him. Marguerite was leaving on her wedding journey, to marry Emmanuel Philibert, Prince of Savoy. (88) A century later, we hear of a prince of Savoy with the same name, who was deaf. Could the handicap have been hereditary in the family, and partially account for the young princess' interest in an old deaf poet? We can only conjecture.

---

[a] Vraiment, ce petit cadet, de médiocre maison, mais qui a eu se faire aimer et estimer des plus puissants personages, peut aspirer aux plus hautes fortunes, êtres courtisan, diplomate, ou, à l' exemple de son père, soldat. Mais n'eut-il pas été perdu pour la poésie si un mal terrible ne l'eut tour à coup force de renoncer à de telles carrières?

In 1552, Du Bellay published a poem in which he expressed his bitter grief at his handicap of hearing loss. Later, apparently comforted somewhat by the example of Ronsard, Du Bellay wrote more cheerfully, dedicating a Hymn to Deafness in honor of Ronsard. (88)

The Reformation re-emphasized the individual's responsibility for his own salvation through knowledge as well as faith. The invention of printing and the use of native languages in writing made possible the spread of learning to the common people. But the day was still to come when all this progress could be translated in terms of education for the handicapped.

Chapter 4

Education for the Deaf—Its Beginning

(1500-1600)

> It is Peter of Ponce, who died in 1584, to whom belongs the honor of having created the art of teaching those deaf-mute from birth. [a] (42, p. 307)

So spoke an early historian of the deaf, writing in 1827. Born in 1520, of a noble family, Ponce de Leon interested himself, as a young man, in the education of deaf-mutes. He established a school for them at the monastery of San Salvador, where he taught, according to all accounts, until his death.

The register of deaths of the monastery was quoted by Degérando (French author on history of the deaf), thus:

> In the year 1584, in the month of August, fell asleep in the Lord, Peter of Ponce, benefactor of that house, who, distinguished by eminent virtues excelled especially and obtained in all the world a justified fame for teaching deaf-mutes to talk. [b] (42, p. 309)

[a] C'est à Pierre de Ponce, mort 1584, qu'appartient la gloire d'avoir crée l'art d'instruire les sourds-muets de naissance.

[b] L'an 1584, au mois d'août, s'endormit dans le Seigneur le frère Pierre de Ponce, bienfaiteur de cette maison, qui, distingué par d'eminentes vertus, excella principalementé et obtint dans tout l'univers une juste célébrité en enseignant aux sourds-muets à parler.

The pupils of Ponce de Leon came from the wealthy and noted families of Spain. The best-known among them were two brothers of the Constable of Castile, Francisco and Pedro de Velasco. (8,a) Other authors added a sister to this family group and placed the son of the Governor of Aragon in the same school. (6; 42; 118)

In a legal document concerning the founding of a chapel, found in the archives of the monastery of San Salvador, Ponce de Leon stated:

> With the industry which God has been pleased to give me, I have had pupils who were deaf and dumb from birth, children of great nobles and of men of distinction, whom I have taught to speak, to read, to write, and to keep accounts, to repeat prayers, to serve the Mass, to know the doctrines of the Christian religion, and to confess themselves with the living voice. (42; 118)

Francisco, the elder of the two Velasco brothers, was heir to a marquisate. Apparently he acquired enough usable speech and language to nullify the legal prohibitions against the right to such inheritance for those born deaf and dumb, and to take up the duties and privileges of his heritage, even military duties.

Several men of authority, who were contemporary with Ponce de Leon, included in their writings references to his work in teaching deaf-mutes. The earliest of these was in a manuscript by Lasso, a lawyer of Oña, written in 1550. He discussed the legal questions which arose as a result of the successful acquisition of speech by these young deaf noblemen, who were thus placed in a position to claim their inheritance and manage their own affairs. (87) It was his conclusion that the deaf who learn to speak are no longer dumb and should have complete "right of progeniture."

Francisco Valles, a friend of Ponce de Leon and physician to Philip II of Spain, was quoted by Degérando, in his account of his friend's work:

> Peter of Ponce, monk of Saint Benedict, my friend; what a wonderful thing! taught deaf mutes from birth to speak; he used for this no other method than teaching them first to write while showing them with his finger the object which was named by the written characters; then in drilling them to repeat with the vocal organ the words which correspond to these characters. [a] (42)

---

[a] Pierre de Ponce, moine de Saint-Benoit mon ami; chose admirable! enseignait aux sourds-muets de naissance à parler; il n'employait a cet effet d'autre moyen qu'en leur apprenant d'abord à écrire en leur montrant du doigt des objets qui etaient exprimés par des caracteres écrits; ensuite, en les exerçant à répéter, par l'organs vocal les mots qui correspondent à ces caracteres.

Early historians also quoted Ambrose de Morales, historiographer to Philip II (72), who was, according to his own words, a witness to some of these things. In his Antiquites d'Espagnés, he said,

> Peter of Ponce taught deaf-mutes to speak with extraordinary perfection. He is the inventor of the art. He has already instructed in this manner two brothers and a sister of the constable, and is now actually occupied with teaching the son of the Governor of Aragon, deaf-mute from birth like the preceding ones. The most surprising thing in his art is that his pupils all reason very well. I am keeping from one of them, don Pedro de Velasco, brother of the constable, a writing in which he tells me that it is to father Ponce that he is indebted for knowing how to talk. [b] (42, p. 309)

There is also evidence that Ponce de Leon left his own records of his methods and their results. These were lost, possibly in a fire that destroyed the library of his monastery. (8,b)

No mention was made of the use of lipreading by Ponce de Leon and his pupils. It may have been accepted as a natural corollary to their learning to speak. From the accounts given, it is difficult to accept the interpretation of some authorities that Ponce de Leon communicated with his pupils by means of conventional signs. (8,b; 75) It seems much more likely that he simply "showed with his finger" by pointing to the object whose name he was teaching at the moment.

The strangest thing about the story of Pedro de Ponce de Leon is that, in spite of all his success and the favorable publicity given to his work, at his death it seemed to die with him.

However, there is some record of another case at about the same time, in the Electorate of Brandenburg, Germany. The Provost of Brandenburg, Joachim Pascha, had a daughter, "who was robbed of her hearing the first year of her life by illness." It grieved her father much that his beloved child should grow up without learning. So, "in the stillness of his study, the holy man worked with a deaf-mute child who was dear to his heart."

He taught her first by means of pictures, and when this did not give her oral speech, it gave him the idea of teaching her written speech, "by which means he not only cultivated his daughter's

---

[b] Pedro de Ponce enseigna aux sourds-muets à parler avec une perfection rare. Il est l'inventeur de cet art. Il a déjà instruit de cette manière deux frères et un soeur du connétable, et s'occupe actuellement de l'instruction du fils du gouverneur d'Aragon, sourd-muet de naissance comme les precedens. Ce qu'il y a de plus surprenant dans son art c'est que ses élèves tout en raisonnent très bien. Je conserve de l'en d'eux, don Pedro de Velasco, frere du connetable, un escrit dans lequel il me dit c'est au père Ponce qu'il a l'obligation de savoir parler.

spirit but placed her in communication with her environment."

Unfortunately, there was no successor to Pascha's work. (134)

One of the next figures to come on the scene of the education of the deaf was Juan Martin Pablo Bonet, born in Torres de Berrellén, Spain, baptized the seventh of January, 1579. (127)

He was a soldier, but also, more particularly, "a man of letters, intelligent and studious." [a] These qualities caught the attention of Juan Fernández de Velasco, who was then the Constable of Castile. In 1607, he took the young man into his service, where he gave such good satisfaction that, upon the death of the constable in 1613, he was retained by the widow as secretary for the new constable, don Bernardino Fernandez de Velasco, a child of four years of age.

The young duchess doña Juana de Córdoba, was left with three children, Bernardino, aged four, Luis, aged three, and a daughter, Mariana, who was a little more than a year old. The second son, Luis, had lost his hearing at the age of two years, during an illness, and "forgetting, little by little, his beginning use of speech, finally became definitely deaf-mute." [b] (127, p. 5)

The chief concern of the widowed mother was to find some help for her little son's misfortune. It was told in the family that, forty years before, deaf brothers of the old constable, grandfather of Luis, had been taught to speak and write by the skill of a monk of Oña, called Pedro de Ponce de Leon. This was considered a marvelous thing, which was also noted in the books of Ambrose de Morales. But it was judged to be a special gift from heaven, rather than the fruit of the good friar's ingenuity, and no one had attempted to continue the work.

Bonet, moved by his obligation to the family and by the immense concern of the young mother, set himself to find out how help could be obtained. His search led him to Manuel Ramírez de Carrión, who was at Montilla, engaged in teaching speech to the deaf Marquis de Priego. At first, the Marquis refused to part with his teacher and secretary. But the influence of powerful friends finally prevailed, and he consented to lend de Carrión to little Luis for three or four years.[a] (127)

Ramírez de Carrión came to Madrid in 1615, and took charge of the boy's education. He was evidently a bright little boy, and it was recorded that he made surprising progress. De Carrión reported

---

[a] un hombre de letras inteligente y estudioso.

[b] olvidando poco a poco el incipiente uso de la palabra, vino a quedar definitivamente sordomudo.

[a] The comment by Ewing that this was the young deaf man taught by Ponce de Leon is evidently inaccurate (54,b).

that, when he had learned to speak, Luis used to say, "I'm not mute, only deaf." [b]

In 1619, Ramírez de Carrión, having used up his leave of absence, returned to the Marquis de Priego at Montilla. Bonet, who had studied the procedures of the boy's tutor, offered his services to the duchess to continue the lad's education.

It has been stated the Ramírez de Carrión was deaf-mute himself. The accounts of his work make this scarcely credible. (54,b)

The statement of some authors that Ramírez de Carrión came after Juan Pablo Bonet seems to have been in error. (20, p. 376; 168,c)

In 1620, Bonet published, at Madrid, his famous book "Reduction de las Letras Y arte para Enseñar a Hablar Los Mudos." [c]

Nowhere in his book did Bonet make any reference to either Ponce de Leon or Ramírez de Carrión, but presented himself as the originator of the method he described. At least one writer felt that Bonet might have made this statement in good faith, knowing little or nothing of Ponce de Leon's work, and having altered and expanded de Carrión's until it became his own. (34)

The book consisted of two parts. Part I was a description of the phonetic qualities of the letters of the alphabet, as contrasted to their names. By associating the letters directly with their phonetic elements, Bonet hoped to simplify reading for the deaf.

Part II described Bonet's philosophy as to methods of teaching the deaf to speak. He advocated, first, the teaching of a one-handed manual alphabet, using pictures illustrating the position of the hand for each letter in association with the printed symbol of the letter, both capital and ordinary forms, written above it. He also insisted that everyone living in a house with a deaf-mute should be forced to learn this manual alphabet.

After the letters were learned in this visual fashion, the pupil was then taught to sound each letter vocally, beginning with the vowels. A chapter of the book dealt with the positions of the speech organs necessary for the proper pronunciation of the speech sounds. Then the pupil was taught syllables, following certain set rules, and after that words, first of one syllable containing two letters each. The first words were to be names of objects at hand, which could be shown him, so that he could associate them directly with their names. When he had achieved some vocabulary in this fashion, he was then taught the Spanish language by grammatical

[b] Yo no soy mudo, sino sordo.
[c] Simplification of Sounds and the Art of Teaching the Dumb to Speak.

steps, which were laid out in order.

In chapter 22, Bonet advocated that

> in order that the deaf-mute may become intelligent and capable, it will be an important part of his education that he be asked every evening what he has done in the daytime. (22, p. 268)

The first recorded comment we have on lipreading was made by Bonet in the last chapter of his book:

> For the deaf-mute to understand what is said to him by the motions of the lips and tongue there is no teaching necessary. . . . Some of these he knows already from learning to speak. . . . It would be an unwarrantable thing to expect all who speak to the deaf to do so with the mouth widely opened. . . . The reduction of the motions to a system to enable the deaf-mute to understand by the lips alone, as it is well known many of them have done, cannot be performed by teaching, but only by great attention on their part; and it is to this that their skill is attributed and not to the skill of the master. (22)

By this time Bonet was forty-one years old, married, and with a son of his own. The Constable Bernardino de Velasco was eleven. Bonet seemed to feel that there was little chance for further advancement in glory or money in the household of Castile. With the consent of the duchess, he transferred his services to the Count of Monterrey. (127)

Young Luis continued to attract attention by his extraordinary achievements, as he grew to manhood. He managed the business affairs of the palace and carried on correspondence with learned people. He seemed to be a favorite of Philip IV of Spain, who gave him, in 1628, the title of Marquis de Fresno.

It was in the court of King Philip that Luis de Velasco encountered Prince Charles of England. James I hoped to unite England and Spain in a pact of peace, after the disastrous Thirty Years War, by the marriage of his son to the Infanta of Spain. In 1623, Charles, the Prince of Wales, and the Duke of Buckingham made the trip to Madrid to pay court to the Spanish princess. In their train was Sir Kenelme Digby, who, having some influence with the Archbishop of Toledo, was invited to join the royal party for the journey. Charles did not marry the daughter of Philip, but he found other things at the court of Spain to draw his interest. (45,b)

He was fascinated by the young deaf lord, who was so accomplished in spite of his handicap. He apparently spent considerable time with Luis de Velasco. Sir Kenelme Digby heartily shared the prince's interest, and later recounted the event in a book he wrote for his son.

He described the young man as

> so deaf that if a gun were shot off close to his eare he could not heare it, and consequently he was dumb.

He also remarked that

> the loveliness of his face and especially the exceeding life and spiritfulness of his eyes and the comeliness of his person and whole composure of his body throughout were pregnant signs of a well-tempered mind within.

Physicians and surgeons had long employed their skill to remedy the handicap, but all in vain.

> At the last, there was a priest who undertook the teaching of him to understand others when they spoke, and to speake himself that others might understand him, for which attempt at first he was laughed at, yet after some years he was looked upon as if he had performed a miracle.
>
> In a word, after strange patience, constancy, and paines, he brought the young lord to speake as distinctly as any man soever; and to understand so perfectly what others said that he would not lose a word in a whole day's conversation. (45,a)

Was this "priest" Juan Pablo Bonet? For Digby went on to say:

> They who have a curiosity to see by what steps the master proceeded in teaching him may satisfie it by a book which he himself hath writ in Spanish on that subject, to instruct others how to teach deaf and dumb persons to speake.

Digby related further that

> he could converse currently in the light, though they he talked with whispered never so softly. And I have seen him, at the distance of a large chambere's breadth, say words after one, that I standing close by the speaker could not heare one syllable of. But if he were in the dark, or if one turned his face out of his sight, he was capable of nothing one said.

Of his speech, Digby said,

> It is true, one great misbecomingnesse he was apt to fall into, whiles he spoke: which was an uncertainty in the tone of his voice; for not hearing the sound he made when he spoke, he could not steadily governe the pitch of his voyce, but it would be sometimes higher, sometimes lower, though for the most part, what he delivered together, he ended in the same key as he began it. (45,a)

This all reads like a familiar story to those of us who are accustomed to similar success with young deaf people orally taught today. But no more than half a century later, the art of teaching oralism to deaf children was again so completely lost that the veracity of this eyewitness account was seriously questioned.

George Dalgarno, the Scot, in 1680, referred to Digby's account of "the young Spanish lord," and commented that, no doubt the priest who was his tutor stood quietly by to cue the young man with secret manual signs. (41,a)

About this same time, there was a physician from Avignon, named Pietro di Castro, who was first physician to the duke of Mantua, Italy. This man took an interest in deaf children, from a physician's point of view. For a time, he accepted Judaism, and adopted the name Ezechielle di Castro. (56) It was under this name that he included a tract entitled "Colostro" (Mothers' Milk) in a medical book about childen's diseases, called "La Commare" (The Midwife).

In this tract, he stated that there was a means of "curing" children who were deaf-mute, so that, while they were still deaf, they were no longer mute but able to speak. This, he admitted, was almost miraculous, but could be accomplished with ingenuity, and he knew of many children in Spain who had been so taught. He himself, he said, had treated the son of Prince Thomas of Savoy, the Marquis of Priego, and the Marquis of Fresno, brother of the Constable of Castile. These young men could now speak without difficulty. He also knew of many others, not of royal families, who had accomplished the same thing.

He stated that he had learned this skill from the man who invented it, Emmanuel Ramírez de Carrión. It was, he said, a rare secret, which he was not ready to disclose now, but would describe in a later lecture. [a] (33,b)

The promised description of his method does not seem to appear in his published works. But other historians have described what they thought was his technique. First, the deaf-mute was to purge himself with hellebore. Then the hair on the crown of his head was shaven, and a salve was applied. This salve was composed of saltpetre, nitre, almond oil, brandy, and naptha, and was to be applied at night. In the morning it was washed off and his hair was combed. When one spoke strongly, then, to the crown of his head, he could perceive voice, and so learn to speak. One writer suggested

[a] Translated from the Italian by Dorothy Sullian, Armed Forces Library, Cleveland, Ohio.

that this "remedy called marvelous" was invented by Ramírez de Carrión especially for the use of Pietro di Castro. (42; 72; 168, c)

We are left to wonder whether Ramírez de Carrión was trying to deceive the doctor, or whether Pietro di Castro was trying to mystify a wondering public concerning the secret of giving intelligible speech to those who could not hear.

It was said that the son of Prince Thomas of Savoy, who was named as one of the pupils of both de Carrión and di Castro, was called Emmanuel Philibert of Carignan, Carignan being a dependency of Savoy. (102)

Spain gave us the beginning of the first systematic language teaching for deaf children. But since universal education of any kind was still far from reality, these earliest teachers seemed to work in isolation, without reference to each other. Yet the teaching situations were ideal for best results. Each teacher had a few children, from the most cultured and intelligent families. He was well-paid to devote his whole attention to the education of these children over a period of years. It is scarcely surprising that the success of these pupils was outstanding.

Chapter 5

A Transition Period

(1600-1650)

The beginning of the seventeenth century was a growing change in the standards and purposes of education. Schools were becoming more and more the responsibility of civil organizations. Much was written and published concerning the philosophy of education. Men had turned away from the dictates of the past, and were exploring eagerly among the possibilities in education and science. They were beginning to look toward universal education as a means of resolving the troubles of the world.

John Amos Comenius (1592-1671) was one of the greatest of those who concerned himself with the education of children at this time. His basic philosophy was that things must come before words, and that symbols are of little use until the child has first had the experience which the symbols represent. He also advocated teaching the whole before its parts. Comenius was so much ahead of the thinking of his time that his teachings had little direct influence on the schools of his own day.

John Locke (1632-1704) urged the training of the senses as the primary step in education. Francis Bacon (1561-1626) advocated the use of experimentation. Scientific discoveries, such as the circulation of the blood by Dr. William Harvey (1578-1657), emphasized the practical value of these philosophies.

Realism was coming to the fore as the basic principle of learning. (38; 48; 95)

These trends were early reflected in the medical writings concerning the deaf. Among the first of these writings was a monograph written by Salomon Alberti, of Nuremburg, Germany, published in 1591 under the title *Oratio de Surditate et Mutitate*. [a]

Alberti commented that the fact that our "ears capture speech" is the basis of the difference between human society and brutes. He discussed the comments of both Aristotle and Hippocrates on the relationship between deafness and lack of speech, adding that, in his opinion, too much authority was attached by later philosophers to these rather casual remarks.

He related instances where muteness was not the result of deafness, since the individuals were able to understand speech and follow a trade, although they could not speak. He mentioned Athos, the son of Croesus, who was mute from infancy. As a young man, he went with his father into battle. When he saw an enemy soldier about to strike his father down, he cried out, "O man, do not kill Croesus!" After this he could speak.

He also called attention to those individuals who could hear a loud sound, and called them hard of hearing rather than deaf.

Alberti suggested that deafness might be due to some lack in the development of the fetus, but went no further in an attempt to elaborate this theory.

He mentioned, with admiration, those who seemed to understand by watching the speaker closely. He thought this must be a very difficult skill, since many sounds are in the back of the mouth and cannot be seen. (4)

The hereditary character of deafness was illustrated by Johannes Schenck (1531-1598) in his description of a family which had several children born deaf. He also attributed it to an embryonic deficiency, without any further explanation.

Among other causes for deafness, he related an instance of a woman whose husband boxed her ears, after which she was deaf. (114)

Another physician who was particularly interested in diseases of the ear was Felix Platter (1530-1614).

His father lacked an education and resolved that his sons should have the opportunity that he had missed. Felix was sent to medical school, November 4, 1552, where he did well. He received his degree as a doctor, September 20, 1557, at Basel, Switzerland, the town of his birth. (105,d)

---

[a] Speaking of Deafness and Dumbness.

Platter made a careful study of anatomy, which he accomplished by means of post-mortem examinations. His books were filled with plates of intricate illustrations of the structures of the human body. One gave a detailed study of the bones of the ear. Another showed the nerves leading to the tongue and the ear, which Platter considered branches of the same nerve in the brain. (105,a)

He also commented on the phenomenon of the conduction of sound through the bones of the head.

Platter stated that the deaf were always mute if the deafness existed from birth, but those who could hear a little, and those who were deafened later in life, could sometimes speak. He said that the cause of deafness was sometimes in the brain and sometimes in the cavity of the ears. If it was in the brain, there was no cure.

He also mentioned the presence of tinnitus, or noises in the ears in many deaf people, and commented on how much this contributed to their confusion in hearing. (105b,c)

Numerous allusions to the deaf and their problems were found in many of the medical and philosophical writings of the day. The air of mystery that seemed to be a part of the double affliction of the deaf, as well as the growing confidence in the powers of education and science, made them most interesting subjects for speculation. (20)

Parallel with the aroused interest in medical research, there grew up a considerable body of speculation and philosophy concerning the fundamental nature of language and speech. Some of these were purely philosophical studies, often with illustrations from the language difficulties peculiar to the deaf. Others had their interest drawn to the deaf, and attempted to construct logical arrangements of language structures that could be used, theoretically, for their instruction. Many were based on long-known manual alphabets and sign languages used by monastic orders under vows of silence, by thieves for secret communication, and in children's games.

One of these frequently referred to by later authors was a treatise called *Of the Art of Signs,*[a] by Giovanni Bonifacio, in 1616. The writer was not interested particularly in the deaf but remarked, at one point, on the extent to which they developed visible language by making signs with their hands. (23; 135)

Not all the writings at this time were concerned with manual languages. P. Francesco Lana-Terzi, a Jesuit of Brescia, Italy, planned a great work of research into the mysteries of nature. In 1670, he published a resumé of the projected work, which he called

[a] De L'Arte des Signes.

Prodromo. (86) His theory was that the deaf pupil should be made examine the positions of the speech organs for each sound, as his teacher spoke them, then imitate them himself. When he could both lipread and imitate the sounds, they were to be assembled into words, and the corresponding objects pointed out to him. (42)

A minister, G. Burnet, traveling through the various countries of Europe, wrote letters home to a friend, describing the things he considered noteworthy on his travels. In the fourth letter, written from Rome, December 8, 1685, he told an appealing story of the fifteen-year-old daughter of a minister at Geneva, Switzerland.

The child had used a few baby words at a year of age, but did not advance beyond that. When she was two, her family discovered she was deaf. She could hear "great noises," but not speech.

The writer said,

> But this child hath, by observing the motion of the mouths and lips of others acquired so many words, that out of these she has formed a sort of jargon, in which she can hold a conversation whole days with those who can speak her own language. (30, p. 203)

She could comprehend some words, but not whole sentences, and at night the family had to light a candle in order to talk with her. Her sister understood her best, and the two could converse at night by touch, for short, simple things.

The Rev. Burnet was much impressed by the "natural sagacity" of the girl. (30)

A small treatise, called *The Deaf and Dumb Man's Discourse,* was published in 1670, by George Sibscota. It was, in reality, a translation of an essay written fifteen years earlier, by Anthony Deusing, professor of medicine at Groningen, Netherlands. (8,b)

The author began by referring not only to the diseases that afflict the human being after birth, but also discussed factors that can cause damage to a child before birth, so that he is already handicapped when he is born. He commented on the opinions of previous writers, such as Aristotle, particularly with reference to the question whether those that are born deaf are dumb also. His opinion was that they were not dumb of necessity. As proof he cited the work of

> one Peter Pontius,[a] a monk of the order of Saint Benedict, and his friend, (who) taught those that were born deaf to speak, by no other way than instructing them first to write, pointing at those things with his fingers that were signified by those characters, and then putting them forward to that motion of the tongue that did correspond to the characters. (115, p. 18)

[a] Pedro de Ponce de Leon.

It was his theory, based in part on a previous discussion by Laurentius, that there is a conjunction of the auditory nerves and the nerves of the tongue, so that if the auditory nerve is damaged, some of this damage is transmitted to the nerves of speech, making articulation difficult.

> And from this Communion of the Vessels proceeds the sympathy between the Ear, the Tongue, and Larynx, and the very affection of the parts are easily communicated one with another.
> . . . and that is the reason most deaf men, at least those whose deafness ariseth from the ill-affection of the nerves of the fifth pair, are Dumb, or else speak with great difficulty. (119, p. 28)

He also described conductive deafness, and thought that the Eustachian tube was the "conduit pipe" by which we heard our own voices with our ears stopped, or music, when we held a stick in our teeth and touched a musical instrument.

He felt very strongly that those born deaf were responsible for learning what they could by sight, and so develop the natural reason that was theirs. (119)

Many more such references were scattered through the literature of the times, testifying to the growing interest in the deaf, and in the general subject of language and communication. Only three more of them need to concern us here, namely, Bulwer of England, Dalgarno of Scotland, and Van Helmont of Germany.

John Bulwer was an English physician, who took an unusual interest in language and its development. In 1644, he published a work called *Chirologia,* or *The Natural Language of the Hand,* and another called *Chironomia,* or *The Art of Manual Rhetoric.* (28,a,b) He analyzed, in these treatises, the application of manual expression in the art of oratory and acting. He was convinced that the "language of the hand" was the one language that was natural in all men. This led him to a study of the means of communication used by deaf persons. He described in some detail the case of a deafened man, Master Babington of Burntwood, who had become so proficient in the use of a manual alphabet, "contryved on the joynts of his fingers," that his wife could converse with him easily, even in the dark.

In 1648, Bulwer published his famous *Philocophus,* or *The Deafe and Dumbe Man's Friend,*

> Exhibiting the Philosophical Verity of that Subtile Art, which May Enable One with an Observant Eie to Heare what Any Man Speaks by the Moving of his Lips. Upon the Same Ground with the Advantage of an Historicall Exemplification apparently Proving that a Man Born

> Deafe and Dumbe may be taught to Heare the Sound of Words with his Eie, and Thence Learn to Speak with his Tongue. (28,c)

The involved title almost describes the book. It was dedicated to Sir Edward Gostwicke and his brother, William, who were deaf, and apparently proficient in signs, but "earnestly desired to unfold your lips" and learn to speak, "accounting your dumbness to be your greatest unhappiness."

Bulwer began to explore the possibility of finding a means to answer this need, when

> coasting along the borders of gestures and voluntary motion I discovered a community among the senses.

By the substitution of one sense for another, Bulwer thought it quite possible for deaf-mutes to learn lipreading and speech, although he favored signs and manual alphabets as a more practical means of communication for them. He even hoped to establish an "academie" for the deaf, in which these new arts of communication could be taught. The hope seems to be as far as he ever went with his Academie.

The first chapter of the book described the organs of speech and their use in articulation, along with fantastic accounts of infants that spoke at birth or soon afterwards. The chapters followed each other with lucid descriptions of the anatomy of the speech organs and their specific movements for each element of speech sounds. Bulwer commented particularly on the fact that speech is movement rather than position. He commented also on the common use of lipreading among hearing persons, describing the gentlemen who came to church and, finding it so crowded that they could not get near the preacher, took spy glasses from their pockets and looked at him through the spy glasses in order to hear him better.

The second part of the book was occupied with a history of deaf and dumb people, and in investigating various causes for deafness. Bulwer made the statement that "men naturally (i.e. born) deaf never learn speech without a teacher." He was intrigued by Sir Kenelme Digby's account of the achievements of the Spanish lord in speech and lipreading, and spent considerable space in discussing the case.

Bulwer's *Philocophus* has been given considerable acclaim as the first English work treating at length the subject of deafness and its accompanying language problems. There is no indication that it had any practical application, then or later, in actually teaching deaf persons.

Another of the theorists on language and communication for the deaf was **George Dalgarno** from Aberdeen, Scotland. He was master of a private grammar school in Oxford, England, for thirty years, and was also master of Elizabeth School in Germany for some time. He died of a fever on August 28, 1687, "aged 60 or more." (41,c)

In 1661, Dalgarno published the *Art of Communication, (using) A Universal Letter Common to All and Philosophical Speech.* [a]

This was apparently an attempt at a universal language. It was a methodical classification of ideas represented by written characters, with no reference to the words of any particular language.

This study of the problem of universal communication led Dalgarno to an interest in the communication problems of the deaf. Twenty years later, in 1680, he published the *Didascalocophus,* or The Deaf and Dumb Man's Tutor. In this book, Dalgarno discussed in great detail his theories concerning the best techniques for teaching language to deaf persons. He compared their situation to that of the blind, and decided that both were entirely capable of learning adequate language skills, if properly taught.

He had no doubt that deaf persons could be taught to speak and lipread. He felt, however, that writing and a form of manual alphabet, which he called dactylology, was more practical for the most part.

He advocated that this language teaching be approached in the same way as one normally learns his mother tongue. Instead of speaking to her deaf child, he advised the mother to spell to him continually on her fingers, and point to the objects she named. He commented that the deaf baby could learn as readily in his cradle as any other,

> if the mother or nurse had but as nimble a hand as commonly they have a tongue. (41,b, p. 118)

Dalgarno warned against too grammatical an approach in teaching language to a deaf pupil, maintaining that

> it is the frequency of recognizing words and using them upon all occasions that makes a man master of a language. (41,b, p. 127)

His manual alphabet was described in Chapter VIII of Ars Signorum. It consisted of placing the letters of the alphabet in various positions upon the inner face of the left hand, in this fashion:

[a] Ars Signorum, Vulgo Character Universalis Et Lingua Philosophica.

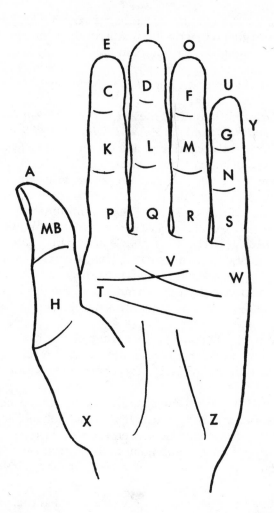

The rules of practice are two: 1. Touch the places of the vowels with a cross touch with any finger of the right hand. 2. Point to the consonants with the thumb of the right hand.

There was also a way of abbreviating double consonants by joining the thumb and finger to point to both at once. (41,b, p. 150)

Dalgarno suggested that a handbook of the finger alphabet be placed on the back of the Horn Book used for teaching letters to hearing children. (41)

Little notice was taken of Dalgarno's work in his own time, and there is no evidence that he ever tried to put it into practice himself.

The **Baron Van Helmont** was the son of a Belgian chemist. He followed his father's profession to some extent, but was much more interested in the occult and mystic things which were still a part of such science in those days. He became particularly interested in a philosophical study of language believing that such study would lead him to great truths. (8,b; 75)

He was persuaded that a language natural to all men must exist, and believed that this language was Hebrew. In 1667, in Sulzbach, Germany, he published a book which he called *Alphabeti vere naturalis Hebraici brevissima delineatio* (a brief description of the actual, natural Hebrew language). It was his idea that each written character of the Hebrew alphabet was shaped after the positions the speech organs took in pronouncing the sound. This he attempted to prove by a curious set of copperplate engravings, in which he showed, within a sectional figure of a man's head, his concept of the positions of the speech organs, with the corresponding Hebrew character written below. (131)

By using these natural speech positions, he stated that he had been able to teach a deaf-mute to speak and answer questions orally in a period of three weeks' time. (8,b; 42)

This claim has been seriously doubted by most authorities, but one author speculated that if his pupil was a child recently deafened by fever, Van Helmont might have simply helped to restore a faculty of speech that would have returned in any case. Since he could not know this, he would have been entirely sincere in his belief that his efforts at teaching had brought about the desired result. (75)

Joseph Degérando, on the other hand, continued with Van Helmont's story, that his pupil learned Hebrew readily, without a teacher. After having learned to read and combine letters, he simply compared the texts of the German and Hebrew Bibles (42, p. 329), and so taught himself Hebrew.

Nothing further seems to have come of Van Helmont's theory during his time. Centuries later, Goldstein (59,b) posed an interesting question as to whether the relationship of the anatomical outlines of speech to the shape of the letter might have been a starting point for the thinking of Alexander Melvill Bell, father of Alexander Graham Bell, which culminated in his Visible Speech Symbols.

Two more men of England not only published treatises on speech and language, in relation to teaching deaf persons, but also made personal application of their own theories. These men were John

Wallis and William Holder, both Fellows of the Royal Society.[a] In spite of the considerable publicity that attended their efforts, there is a good deal of contradiction in the details of the historical accounts that have been left to us. The important facts, however, seem to be clear.

John Wallis was born in 1616 at Ashford, Kent in England. He was a mathematician, and in 1649 he was awarded the Chair of Geometry at Oxford. (75)

In 1653, he published his *Grammatica Linguae Anglicanae cui praefigitur De Loquela Sive Sonorum Formationes,*[b] usually called *De Loquela.*

This work was popular enough to be published in a number of editions. The fourth edition came out in 1674. In the fifth edition, which was not dated, Wallis added a paragraph to the effect that not only foreigners but also stammerers and deaf persons could be taught to speak English clearly by his method. (166)

The *De Loquela* described in analytical fashion the speech elements, arranged according to the position of the speech organs in their utterance. (133)

As a result of his published interest in the deaf, Wallis was asked to undertake the education of Daniel Whaley, of Northampton, a young man of twenty-five, who had been deaf since the age of five. He had, after the illness that took his hearing, lost his speech, not all at once, but by degrees, over a period of half a year.

Our knowledge of the techniques Wallis used in teaching his pupil is gathered largely from letters he wrote to friends, which were later published in several technical journals of the day. In a year's time, Wallis stated, he had successfully taught this young man to speak intelligibly and to read and write the English language.

He gave this account of the young man's accomplishments:

> The Person to whom the foregoing Discourse doth refer is Mr. Daniel Whaley, son of Mr. Whaley, late of Northampton. He was present at the Meeting of the Royal Society, May 21, 1662, and did there, to their great satisfaction, pronounce distinctly enough such words as by the Company were proposed to him; and though not altogether with the usual tone or accent, yet so as to be easily understood. About the same time also (his Majesty having heard of it, and being willing to see him) he did the like several times at Whitehall in the Presence of his Majesty,

[a] The Royal Society was an academy of scientists and philosophers organized for the licensing of books and promoting knowledge. The first such organization in England was under King James in 1616. The present Royal Society was chartered in 1662.
[b] Grammar of English for Foreigners with an Essay on Speech or the Formation of Sounds.

his Highness Prince Rupert, and divers others of the Nobility. In the
Space of a year, which was the whole time of his Stay with Dr. Wallis,
he had read over a great part of the English Bible, and had attained so
much   Skill   as   to   express   himself   intelligibly   in
ordinary Affairs, though not elegantly, yet so as to be understood.
(161, pp. 392-393)

Wallis began his teaching of Daniel Whaley by making use of the
gestures the young man had developed for communication. From
this he proceeded to the written alphabet, then to a manual
alphabet proposed by Dalgarno. (75) Articulation, he taught
separately, following his own principles of speech sounds as out-
lined in his *De Loquela*. For language teaching, he set up grammatical steps in logical order, arranging nouns by classes, and proceed-
ing through parts of speech syntax. The pupil kept a growing book
of his own home-made dictionary and grammar, as his work progressed. (161; 187,a,b)

After his first two pupils, Wallis abandoned the use of articulation, as taking more time and effort than it was worth, and used
reading, writing and a manual alphabet entirely. (8,b)

That Wallis and Dalgarno were acquainted is evident by reference
made to the work of "my good friend Dr. Wallis" by Dalgarno in
The Deaf and Dumb Man's Tutor. (41,b) Arnold (8,b) stated that
Wallis, by his own account, had never seen Bonet's work, but
Hodgson (75) reported that Wallis was in correspondence with
Digby and through him familiar with the work of Bonet.

Dr. William Holder, born in the same year as Wallis, was primarily interested in music. In 1659, while he was Rector of
Bletchington, he was requested to undertake the teaching of Alexander Popham, the son of Admiral Popham and Lady Wharton, who
had been born deaf and was at that time ten or eleven years old.

This he did and became so interested in the work that he wrote
an account of his methods and philosophy, which he published ten
years later, under the title of *Elements of Speech*. (77)

In the preface of this book, he expressed his surprise that the
alphabets of all languages were not all alike and arranged in some
logical order of sound production.

The Consequences whereof have been to render Languages more difficult to be learnt, and needlessly to advance Orthography into a
troublesome and laborious Art and to hide the Nature of Letters in
obscurity. . . .
    And it having happened to me, some years past, to have been deeply
engaged in this same consideration of the Alphabet, by a Worthy

Design of giving Relief to à Deaf and Dumb Person, in the year 1659, recommended to my Care: and being at last prevailed with by divers Persons, who remember the success of that Enterprise to Communicate the Way and Method I then used; I have ventured to publish my thoughts concerning the Nature of Letters.

Holder analyzed in precise detail the positions of the speech organs in the pronunciation of speech elements. He arranged the sounds in the order of what he called the "appulse" of one organ upon another, and suggested the order of presentation to be used in teaching these sounds to a deaf child. Sounds were to be taught individually, then combined into syllables, and the syllables into words, which were then associated with the objects they represented.

It is said that Holder used a tongue-shaped leather thong to show his young pupil how to place his tongue. (75, p. 102)

He discussed the substitution of sight for hearing, and felt that writing should be taught first, so that the pupil might at once associate the sound he learned with the written symbol and so help his memory to retain it. He was convinced of the merit of his method and stated that

the chief design here intended by this account of the Natural Alphabet is to prepare a more easie and expedite way to instruct such as are Deaf and Dumb, and Dumb only by consequence of their want of hearing . . . to be able to pronounce all Letters and Syllables and Words and in good measure discern them by the Eye, when pronounced by another. (77, p. 15)

He added also,

And by these ways (as I myself have made some experiment) it is not impossible, no, nor very difficult to be done even for those who are born Deaf and Dumb. (77, p. 16)

In the appendix to his book, Holder went more fully into his own theories concerning hearing and speech:

Amongst Dumb Persons there are very few who are such through defect in the Organs of Speech; but most commonly that Imperfection is the effect, or rather consequence, of want of Hearing, by some defect in the Organs appertaining to that sense. (77, p. 111)

He felt that hearing loss was due to a lack of proper tension in the drum membrane of the ear, perhaps by some irregularity of the bones of the middle ear, or defect in the muscles of that area. This

he proved to his own satisfaction by the experiment of beating a
drum behind his pupil, in order that the vibration might tighten the
tympanic membrane. At such times, he said, the boy could hear his
name spoken softly behind him, although he could hear nothing
otherwise. He also related similar circumstances of a deaf gentleman
who could understand only when he was in a coach that was rumbl-
ing noisily over a cobblestone street.

Holder seems to have been a gentle and understanding teacher.
He frequently cautioned against forcing the pupil to tasks that were
too difficult for him. He said it was irksome for a deaf person to
exert his voice, and that he was soon subject to weariness in the
lungs and larynx, so that it was hard to make him work. He advised
that he should be

> gently and discreetly treated . . . taking great care that he may not hate
> his task but do it cheerfully.

The lesson exercises should be brief but frequent, and the pupil
encouraged by "much applause and admiration."

Young Alexander Popham was described as having his head and
face distorted, with the right side elevated and the left depressed. In
this condition the left ear was closed while the right ear was
distended. (77, p. 159)

After three years of teaching, the boy seemed to have made small
progress. He could pronounce his own name and some other
words. His mother may have been dissatisfied with his
achievements, for she sent him to Wallis, who was at that time
being very successful in his teaching of Daniel Whaley. (75)
Although Wallis later claimed equal success with Alexander
Popham as he had with his previous pupil, there is no record that he
ever exhibited this boy's accomplishments.

From the description given of young Master Popham, it would
seem probable that he had sustained more damage than a simple
hearing loss, and his lack of achievement may have been due to the
limitations of the pupil rather than to any lack of skill in either of his
teachers.

Holder took offense at Wallis's claims as the first teacher to
describe a successful method for teaching deaf persons, and
claimed this honor for himself. (155,b) Wallis answered with equal
fervor, defending his own priority. (187,a)

Concerning this dispute, we must agree with Hodgson, when he
said,

> Whalley and Popham were the first two children in England to be
> taught, Wallis and Holder the first two teachers, as far as we know, and

theirs the first quarrel. This petty tendency was unfortunately to remain a feature of the work. (75, p. 101)

Realism became the guiding principle in education for this period of history. This philosophy encouraged the use of experimentation and exploration among all natural phenomena, especially those directly related to the welfare of mankind.

Chapter 6

Teaching the Deaf— Becoming a Profession

(1650-1700)

In the previous accounts of teachers who undertook the education of deaf persons, most were isolated cases, with only one or two pupils, and those acquired by some accident not particularly related to the major interest of the teacher. This picture was gradually changing. The education of children was becoming rapidly more widespread and universal. It was a natural corollary that the profession of teaching was attracting more general interest as a means of livelihood, as well as a fascinating source for philosophical speculation.

Those who found some success in the specialized education of the hearing-handicapped adopted it as their profession. Making it also their means of living, most of them shrouded their methods in secrecy. They were living in a sharply competitive age, when the man of modest station had difficulty in maintaining an adequate income for his family unless he possessed a profitable monopoly of some sort.

It is little wonder, and not especially to their discredit, that many of the early teachers of the deaf guarded the secrets of their success with a jealousy that was a common procedure at that time. That this point of view was extremely shortsighted and worked to the disadvantage of the profession cannot be denied. But those were the facts.

Among the most generous and influential of the teachers of the deaf in this period was Johann Konrad Amman. He was born in 1669, in Schaffhausen, Switzerland, where his father officiated as municipal physician and was also professor of Greek and physics at the College. The young man studied medicine at Basel, completing the requirements for his degree as Doctor of Medicine, at the age of eighteen, with a treatise on the inflammation of the lungs.

Following this he made the customary post-graduate journey of observation to other countries. He was so charmed with Holland, according to his own statement (5,a), that he returned in 1690, to settle in Amsterdam.

In addition to his medical practice, Amman seems to have become interested in trying to educate deaf-mutes. One day, Pietar Koolaert, a merchant of Haarlem, walked into Amman's study and heard speech from a girl who was formerly mute. Although skeptical, he was sufficiently impressed to persuade Amman to come to Haarlem and teach his deaf-mute daughter, Esther. (5,a; 85)

Amman was successful enough in this enterprise to be encouraged to publish an account of his work for the benefit of others. His first book, *Surdus Loquens,*[a] written in Latin, appeared in Amsterdam in 1692. Three weeks later, an enlarged edition, *De Doove Sprekende,* was published in Haarlem, dedicated to Koolaert. (85)

Prior to this time, Amman had not known of the work of any other teachers of deaf. The publication of his book soon brought him the comments and criticisms for which he asked. Wallis wrote to him from England. As one result of their correspondence, an English translation of Amman's book appeared in 1694. (85) Van Helmont came to see him. Since they shared a mystical view of the origin of language, the two men must have found much in common. Van Helmont had suspected Amman of copying from his own book, but after seeing him work, he admitted that Amman's methods were original and an improvement on his own. (5,a)

In 1700, Amman published another book which was a much extended version of *Surdus Loquens.* This he called:

> A Dissertation on Speech, in which not only the Human Voice and the Art of Speaking are traced from their Origin But the Means are also described by which Those who have been Deaf and Dumb from their Birth may Acquire Speech and Those who Speak imperfectly may learn how to correct their Impediments. (5,a)

[a] The Speaking Deaf.

The book did just that.

Amman believed that speech was of Divine origin, and so was not only the privilege of all men, but could be achieved by all. Speech was, therefore, the fundamental aim of his teaching.

Amman, himself, had a great deal of faith in his own methods, which seemed to be justified by the results. He stated that he had "failed with only one, a girl whose intellect was dull."

He said,

> First, what I require in teaching a deaf and dumb person is that he shall be of a quick and docile disposition, neither too young nor too advanced in life, but verging on youth, between eight and fifteen years old; and next that his organs of speech shall be perfect. (5,a, p. 91)

Amman described his methods in generous detail. His first concern for a pupil was to have him achieve a good clear voice, and to control it well. He was puzzled as to how his deaf pupils were able to distinguish breath sounds from voiced sounds, although he could see that they were aware of the difference. He soon learned from them that they could feel the vibrations of the voice, and immediately made use of the knowledge by placing their hands on his throat as he taught speech.

He talked to himself in a mirror, and decided from the sight of his own speaking that a deaf person could be taught to speak by visual means. He also had his pupils use mirrors in their speech practice.

He advocated using every response of the pupil to the fullest extent. If a pupil, upon being asked to give a certain sound, gave another by mistake, he was not to be corrected, but shown instead the written symbol for the sound he had made and drilled in its repetition immediately.

The names of the most obvious things were to be taught first, then other parts of speech in the simplest order, using "amusing and useful examples." (5,a)

Lipreading was an obvious part of the language achievements of Amman's pupils. A favorite lesson technique of his was to read with his pupils a few lines from a book. Then they closed their books, while he read to them again the same lines, and they wrote what he dictated.

In the Latin version of his book, Amman said, "Thus with the eyes, as though with the ears, afterward they hear." [a] (5,b)

Amman commented that

---

[a] Tam oculis, quam auribus, postea audient.

if hearing alone were given to one born deaf, either by art or through a miracle, yet he could speak no more than a new-born child, until he had been taught a language. (5,a, p. 51)

He said, with a good deal of charity,

I have often been amused at the absurd opinions of different persons on this subject, who, believing that I infuse Speech into deaf-mutes with a little potion of medicine, complain that I ask too great a fee for curing, . . . and although the method I pursue has nothing miraculous about it, the patience necessary to the practice of it is all but miraculous. (5,a, p. 52)

By his own account, Amman also taught good speech to persons with articulation defects, "speech aphasia," and stammering, using the same principles he used with deaf pupils.

Amman was most generous in sharing with the world the techniques he used in teaching, but few details of his personal life have come down to us. He was married in 1694 to Maria Birrius, and they had at least four children. He died at Warmond, Netherlands, in 1724. His grave-site is not known. (5,b; 122)

Amman's success had a good deal of influence on his contemporaries. In Germany, in particular, his methods took hold in the growing development of the education of the deaf. Many names were mentioned briefly among the writers, physicians, and educators of the time, as concerning themselves in one way or another with the problems of deafness.

One of these, L. W. Kerger, with the help of his sister, established and taught a school in Liegnitz, Silesia, which was reported to be quite successful.

Kerger described his work in a letter he wrote to Ettmüller of Leipzig, April 5, 1704. After discussing briefly the history of the education of the deaf, of which he seemed to know a great deal, he went on to a discussion of his methods and his reasons for them.

He approved of Amman's methods and thought they might be quite practical for the few deaf-mutes one met from well-to-do families. But most of the deaf, he stated, "are poor and in the common houses," and "time fails for my older ones." He, therefore, felt that for them the most practical method was the one that gave them a means of communication with the least expenditure of time and effort. For there was nothing wrong, he said, in the finger art, and nothing intrinsically helpful in printer's ink.

So he advocated the teaching of reading and writing as the simplest, most rapid approach to learning a language, and the use of dramatic pantomime and drawings to give it meaning.

His sister, he said, "who is better at it than I," taught deaf-mute girls to speak, and also their own sister who was deaf and dumb. He thought his own pupils could well have done the same, "if I had more time." (5,a; 42, 83)

Another Silesian, Georg Raphel, was born in Luben, September 10, 1673. He went to school in Hamburg, Germany, where he was also secretary to Professor Placcius. When, in 1696, he enrolled at the University of Rostock, he lived in the home of Professor Fecht, a teacher of theology, at the recommendation and expense of his sponsor in Hamburg. Three years later, Placcius, knowing his death was near, recommended him for a scholarship at the Gymnasium. This Raphel refused, and earned his way by means of several positions. He was magistrate in Rostock and was on call as senior assistant master of the grammar school of Luneburg. He was pastor of the church of St. Nicholas and eventually became superintendent of the same church. He died June 5, 1740. (107)

Of his six children, three daughters were deaf. He educated them all himself, mostly by means of Amman's methods, which he learned when he discovered the need of his eldest daughter. (42)

It is the story of his eldest daughter, Magdlein, and her father's efforts at teaching her that is appealingly told in Raphel's book, *Kunst Taube und Stumme reden zu lehren,* [a] (107) published first in 1718 (8,b, p. 31). It was an effort to make available to other parents of deaf children the methods Raphel found successful with his own.

As he stated, God willed to give him a lovely daughter, intelligent and superior in every way, but totally deaf from birth. She had not been ill, nor had there been any change in her. But at a year of age she still did not respond to her own name when called. Since she was very alert in other ways, this caused her family to wonder. She babbled a great deal, just like other babies, so they thought she would surely begin to talk soon. But when another year had passed and she still could not talk, her parents began to realize that she could not hear. Then they were "in great sorrow," especially since the lack of hearing was not the only problem, but speech was also lacking, since children learn to speak by hearing. (107, p. 36)

Still her father clung to the hope that she would, in time, learn to talk, although he admitted that he had seen people who lost their hearing gradually lose their speech also. The child's continued vocalization included clear syllables, so that at five she could be persuaded to repeat the word "papa," and other simple syllables, on request. But she never used any of these vocalizations with

[a] The Art of Teaching Deaf and Dumb to Speak.

meaning, proving that she did not understand that everything had its own name.

When he finally decided that there was no hope for a recovery of his daughter's hearing, and consequently speech, her father set himself to discover what could be done to teach her. In a Dresden newspaper in 1711, he found an article by Amman, about one Elias Schulze, who was born deaf and dumb, but learned to read within a year's time, being taught by Amman. The author gave a number of proofs of the success of such teaching, and stated that children of eight were ready to begin this sort of education. Raphel also had as witness a merchant of Hamburg, whose deaf son had learned to read, write, and speak.

Raphel resolved immediately that when Magdlein was eight she should be ready to go to Dresden. She was born May 13, 1708, and it was now October, 1715, so he began immediate preparations.

He secured a copy of Amman's tract, which was in Latin, and carefully translated the lessons into German, as he used them with his daughter. He made every effort to arrange the lessons so that the child could learn most easily, and when one method did not work well he would try another.

The child learned rapidly and eagerly, although her father said that, with his busy pastoral duties, he often had to neglect her lessons for weeks at a time. He said her voice was louder than most, and sometimes somewhat muffled and did not ring as clearly as it should, except when she cried; then it was as clear as anyone's.

However, she became very proficient in speech, and was talented and personable in every way. She died at twenty, and was greatly missed. (107) But her father evidently felt that his own teaching was successful enough with her and her two younger sisters that he decided to keep the latter at home.

At about this same time, a pastor named James Wild, of Niederoff, Germany, hired a mechanic of Frankfurt, one Henry Louis Muth, to construct for him a machine that could be made to imitate the movements of the speech organs. Such an apparatus, Wild thought, would be a much better guide for teaching speech to a deaf-mute than the use of a mirror. In spite of its ingenuity, nothing much seems to have come of the idea. (42)

The first of the teachers of the deaf to put his pupils under a bond of secrecy was an Englishman named Henry Baker (1698-1774). They were not to reveal the methods he used to teach them, under penalty of a cash bond of 100 pounds. (75)

Henry Baker was a naturalist and made a name for himself with his use of a microscope, although his business was selling books. At the end of his apprenticeship to the bookseller, in 1720, as a young man of twenty-two, Baker went to Enfield to visit a relative. This relative, John Forster, an attorney, had a daughter Jane, eight years old, who was born deaf. Baker was intrigued by the child and the challenge her problem presented. He wrote,

> Heaven put into my thoughts a method of instructing her to read, write, and understand, and speak the English language. (75, p. 120)

Jane's father begged the young man to stay and make a trial of his ideas. Baker was willing, and remained with the Forster family

> till I had perfected her in the language, and taught her not only to read, write, and speak it readily, but likewise to understand the speech of others by sight, and be able to hold a regular conversation with them upon most subjects. (8,b, p. 38)

Because of his insistence on secrecy, not too much is known about Baker's pupils or his methods. It is said he taught a number of children from wealthy families, with a great deal of success. Samuel Johnson once visited him, and was much impressed by his work. He must have urged Baker to share his technique with the world, because he said later that Baker "once flattered me with the hope of seeing his method published." (80)

In 1927, Baker's daybook was discovered in the archives of the Royal Microscopical Society. This record showed that he taught hearing people with speech defects as well as the deaf. He selected his pupils with care, accepting only those who could profit by his teaching. Hodgson has quoted an item from the daybook, in which Baker noted:

> To teaching Miss Chichester, an almost total want of speech, but not deaf. . . . 27 16s 6d. . . . I found her capacity very defective and declined teaching her anymore. (75, pp. 120-121)

Some of the exercise books used by Baker's pupils have been found. They seem to indicate that his methods were similar to those of Wallis, with a few improvements of his own.

Because of his secrecy, his work had little influence beyond his own pupils.

One who has been called "the greatest teacher of them all" was Jacobo Rodríguez Pereira. He was born at Berlanga, Portugal, on April 11, 1715, in the Spanish Estremadura. His family were Spanish Jews, who had been driven from their own country by persecution, and took refuge in Portugal. They moved from there to Bordeaux, in southern France, in 1741. (117; 8,b)

Pereira took an early interest in teaching deaf persons. A letter he wrote to a friend in 1734, at the age of nineteen, asked for books and information on the subject. Some authorities state that this interest grew from his successful teaching of his own sister, who was a deaf-mute. (8, b, p. 32) An earlier biographer stated that it was unknown how or why he became interested in the deaf. (117)

In 1745, Pereira had achieved enough success with Aaron Beaumain, a deaf boy of thirteen, to warrant his demonstrating his accomplishments before interested persons in La Rochelle. M. d'Azy d'Etavigny, director of five farms at La Rochelle, watched the demonstration with more than casual interest. He had a deaf son, whom the most celebrated doctors in Europe had pronounced incurable.

M. d'Azy d'Etavigny wanted immediately to send his son to Pereira to be educated. Upon investigating he decided that the fees were too high, and tried to find a less expensive method. He bought a copy of Amman's book on teaching the deaf, gave it to two friends who were priests, and told them to educate his son according to the demonstration of Aaron Beaumain.

The two friars read the book, then set themselves to "gesticulate and vociferate" with the boy. They also studied the publications of Wallis and Bonet on the same subject. But after a year they gave it up and advised M. d'Azy d'Etavigny that he had better send his son to Pereira.

He took their advice. He and Pereira drew up and signed a contract that was apparently satisfactory to both. Young d'Etavigny was to be educated by Pereira at a tuition of 3000 libras. One third of this price was to be paid in advance, the second third when the pupil had reached a certain specified level of vocabulary and language accomplishment, and the last third when he had completed his education to the mutual satisfaction of his father and his teacher. (117)

The young man had also some sort of instruction from another deaf aristocrat, Etienne de Fay, who worked as a sculptor in the cathedral of Amiens. He was sixteen when he was referred to Pereira, and had apparently accomplished little that was educationally satisfactory before that time. (42, p. 384)

Even so, in two years his teacher felt that he had made enough progress to demonstrate his accomplishments before the Academy at Caen. This roused so much interest that the Academy of Science[a] at Paris appointed a commission to study the work of Pereira and

[a] The French Academy of Science was an organization of scholars similar to the Royal Society of England.

asked for a demonstration. He appeared before the Academy with d'Azy d'Etavigny, June 11, 1749. b (42)

The commission, headed by the eminent scientist Comte Buffon, reported very favorably on their investigation. They noted that the young deaf student read and pronounced distinctly, that he answered questions very sensibly, both verbally and by writing, and in all ways showed a competent knowledge and skill in the use of language. The witnesses commented that his voice was somewhat rough, but it was their opinion that if deaf children were taught from the age of seven or eight they would do much better in voice quality. (117)

This demonstration before the Academy of Science brought Pereira an introduction to the King, by the Duc de Chaulnes. The duke took a special interest in Pereira, because his young godson, Saboureux de Fontenay, was born deaf and needed a teacher.

As in the case of d'Azy d'Etavigny, young Saboureux had previous teachers. In 1746, at the same time the two priests were struggling to find a teaching technique for d'Etavigny, de Fontenay was receiving some sort of instruction from M. Lucas, "common carpenter from the Ganges," apparently, India. (42, p. 388) What his qualifications were or how he taught seem to have been lost.

At the age of thirteen, Saboureux de Fontenay was added to the list of Pereira's pupils. According to all accounts, he was an excellent student, and went on to distinguish himself in further demonstrations for his teacher. He appeared before the Academy of Science, January 13, 1751. a (42, p. 391) His letters to his friends showed a high degree of culture and learning. He even taught himself a second language. It is also recorded that he later taught several other deaf persons at least the manual part of his own language achievement, with good results.

Pereira was a practical man, and made considerable study of the degrees of deafness. In describing the achievements of de Fontenay, he took care to add,

> We must not neglect to note, however, that young Saboureaux was affected only by a deafness of the second degree. b (42, p. 401)

Of Pereira's methods we have quite a detailed knowledge, gleaned in part from letters and accounts of his pupils, and in part from

b From L'Histoire de l'Academie des Sciences, Anné 1749.

a From L'Histoire de l'Academie des Sciences, Anné 1749, p. 183.

bNous ne devons pas négliger de remarquer encore que le jeune Saboureaux n'était affecté que d'une surdit de second degré.

the report of the Academy of Science. His pupils were placed under an oath of secrecy by Pereira, but apparently had no qualms about telling at least a part of the story after they left the school. A letter written by M. Saboureux de Fontenay on December 26, 1764, described his education in considerable detail. (42, 8,b; 118)

Pereira would accept no more than twelve pupils to work with at one time. (42)

He used a one-handed manual alphabet, in which the position of the fingers was intended to suggest the positions of the speech organs for making that sound. This "alphabet" represented, not letters, but phonic qualities, and was used as an aid to pronunciation. Mimetic signs were allowed only until a more oral means of communication could be established, after which they were abandoned.

For those completely bereft of sound, Pereira substituted the sense of touch for noting the vibrations of the voice, and worked on intonation and accent. Auditory training exercises were used for those who still had some hearing. In these exercises Pereira attempted to sharpen the pupils discrimination of sounds by drill in recognition of various sounds by means of such hearing as remained. Special exercises in sight and touch were designed to train the students to perceive by these means things usually noticed by the ears in hearing people.

Pereira offered two courses. For the poorer and more numerous clients, he gave a short course of fifteen months, which covered the most important of the current necessities of living. Those more favored, who could stay four or five years, were offered a superior course including intellectual and moral rules and methods. (117)

Saboureux de Fontenay had the full course, apparently, for he stayed with Pereira for five years. (8,b)

Pereira must have received a full measure of satisfaction from his life's work. His pupils were successful and famous. He received good fees for teaching them. He was given honor and recognition from the Academy of Science and granted a Royal pension from France. In 1760, he was elected a Fellow of the Royal Society of England. (75) There was not much more that he could have desired in his own lifetime.

After his death, the memory of his work received high praise and honor. His biographer proposed that two of the pillars at the Institution for the Deaf and Dumb in Paris should be inscribed, one with the name of de l'Épée and the other with the name of Pereira. He suggested these inscriptions:

Jacob-Roderíguez Pereira	Carlos-Miguel de l'Épée
Primer Maestro de Sordos y	Primer Director del Instituto
Mudos en Francia	Nacional de Sordos y Mudos
1734—1780	1771—1789[a] (117, p. 230)

He added this comment as proof for his claim to a high place in history for Pereira:

> Those deaf from birth will speak and have as much ability as other men in all that does not depend on hearing.
> There will be no more deaf-mutes. There will be deaf speaking ones.[b] (117)

It was always Pereira's intention that the secret of his success should be known and carried on only by his own family. But he placed such emphasis on secrecy that even his own family did not know his methods.

After Pereira's death, his son tried to revive his father's fame and carry on his work. He failed completely, and died young, leaving his mother and his young widow with two small sons, aged two and six years, without a means of livelihood.

The two women set themselves to rediscover the family secret. They had bright hopes of restoring the family fortunes in time for the little boys to carry on the work in all the glory that had been their grandfather's.

One by one, they looked up old pupils of Pereira's school, but found none that could help. Finally they located an old lady, Madame Marois, who had been a pupil of Pereira in 1756. They traveled to see her. She was their last hope. She could still speak, but she was an octogenarian and becoming senile. The methods by which she had learned had vanished from her memory. (42; 117)

So died with Pereira a work that might have been spread abroad with great advantage for all concerned.

And yet, with the eighteenth century, the work of giving language and education to deaf-mutes began to attain the dignity of a profession. With the rapidly changing developments in all education, the deaf came in for a fair share of interest and attention.

[a]
Jacob Rodrigo Pereira	Charles Michael de l'Épée
First Teacher of Deaf and	First Director of the National
Dumb in France	Institution for Deaf and Dumb
1734-1780	1771-1789

[b] Los sordos de Nacimiento hablarán y se habrán tan capaces como los otros hombres de todo lo que no dependa del oido.
No habrá mas sordomudos. Habrá sordoparlantes.

Chapter 7

Schools for the Deaf— Their Beginnings

(1700-1825)

The eighteenth century and early nineteenth century saw still more basic changes in the philosophy and administration of education. Nations were beginning to waken to public and civic responsibility for the upbringing of children.

In France, this took the form of a closely-organized central authority for education, vested in the state. It eventually came to have great significance in all French education, and particularly in reference to the education of the deaf.

In England, the wealthy and aristocratic classes looked askance at universal education. If the great masses of the common people became educated much beyond the system of practical apprenticeship, they might well present a threat to the position of the aristocracy. But the nobility were not callous to the condition of the over-worked, under-nourished children of the poor, when it was called to their attention. They established charity schools for these children, supported by contributions from wealthy patrons and administered by Boards of Trustees. The schools for the deaf fell inevitably into this same pattern.

Only in Germany did the system of state-supported schools take hold this early in the history of education. Rulers of various German principalities took thoughtful note of the work of individual educators within their territories. If they were found worthy, their schools were taken under state patronage. This also occurred with schools for the deaf.

Of all the names that are prominent in the history of the education of the deaf, one of the best-known in all recent times and in all countries is that of the Abbé de l'Épée. For it was he who first made the education of the deaf a matter of public concern. It was he who first made such education available to the poor.

FRANCE

Charles Michel de l'Épée was born in Versailles, France, November 24, 1712, the son of an architect in the royal service. When as a young man, he developed an interest in religious work, his parents were at first opposed, then yielded to his inclination. He received a good education, and prepared for the priesthood. However, his religious thinking followed the philosophy of the Jansenists, and at that time in the history of France the Jansenists were out of favor. When the young applicant was presented with the formula of faith required in the Paris diocese, he found it contrary to some of his beliefs and refused to sign. This closed the door of the priesthood to him.

He then tried the practice of law, but could not bring himself to be content with it. Of an intensely religious nature, the priesthood was still his chosen work. So he finally signed the required formula. Supported by his uncle, Monseigneur Bossuet, the Bishop of Troyes, who was attracted by his piety and zeal, he was granted a position in the work he loved, and for a time was very happy in it. But when his patron died he found himself again at odds with his religious superiors and deprived of his parish. For twenty-five years, he lived quietly, as an obscure priest. (18, p. 71; 76, p. 6; 168,a)

One day, as he walked the streets of Paris, he chanced to stop at a house, where he found twin sisters at home alone. He spoke to them and was surprised that they gave him no answer. When their mother returned, she informed him with tears that they were deaf-mute. Another priest, Père Vanin, a neighbor of the family, had been attempting to give them some religious instruction by means of pictures. Now that he was dead, they were desolate, because they did not know where else to turn for help. (44,b; 76, p. 6)

(The comment made by Best that the sisters were orphans must have been a misinterpretation.) (20, p. 380)

The good Abbé was much disturbed at the thought that these souls would be lost because they could not know the way to salvation. He immediately decided to undertake their instruction. In the Introduction to his book, he said:

> When I took on the education of the two deaf and dumb twin sisters, it did not enter my head to teach them to speak. Charmed with the facility of teaching them to write, I did not think of untying their tongues. (44,b)

The success de l'Épée had with the two sisters soon attracted more deaf pupils. One day, some strangers, who had come to witness a public lesson, offered de l'Épée a Spanish book they had to sell. At first the Abbé was not interested, because he did not know Spanish. Then he saw that the book contained a beautiful copperplate illustration of the manual alphabet of the Spaniards. The book was Bonet's *Arte para Enseñar a Hablar los Mudos*. De l'Épée bought it, and set himself to learn Spanish in order to read it.

Later someone told him of Amman's book *Dissertatio de Loquela*. He found it in a friend's library and studied that one also. But at the begining of his teaching, he had not been aware of the work of any of his predecessors. His initial techniques were entirely his own. (44,b, pp. 159-161)

From this time on, de l'Épée devoted his life to teaching the deaf. His school grew gradually larger, supported mainly by funds from de l'Épée's own small private income. Soon he began to attract wider notice. Rulers, educators, men of letters came to see his work and were impressed.

Louis XVI, King of France, gave to the school the revenues of a suppressed convent. The Empress Catherine of Russia sent him gifts. The latter he declined, telling the Empress that if she wished to do him a favor, she should send instead a deaf child to be taught or a teacher to be trained.

The Emperor Joseph II of **Austria** came to pay a visit to the school. He had become interested in the plight of a young deaf lady of Vienna. After watching the lessons for two and a half hours, he asked the Abbé what he should do for the young lady's education. De l'Épée suggested two alternatives; either he would teach her himself, if she came to Paris, or, if the Emperor wished to send a suitable candidate, he would train a teacher for him.

He decided to send the Abbé Stork who came bearing a letter from the Emperor, in which he said that, your love for the welfare of humanity makes me hope that you will contribute willingly to extend your charity also for a part of the German deaf and dumb, in training for them a teacher.

De l'Épée was happy to accept the Abbé Stork and found him a ready student. In five months, the young priest was teaching classes, while de l'Épée "sat by, an admiring witness." In three more months, he returned to Vienna, where he opened the first state school for the deaf in 1779.

The one concern of the Abbé de l'Épée was the instruction of as many deaf persons as possible. To him this was especially urgent, since he believed that education for religious instruction was necessary for the salvation of their souls. So he shared freely all he knew, and welcomed all who came to him for training as teachers. (120,b)

In 1776, he published his *Instruction des Sourds et Muets par la Voie des Signes Méthodiques.*[a] This work was greatly expanded and published as a full amount of his method, in 1784, under the title *La Véritable Manière d'Instruire les Sourds et Muets, Confirmé par une Longue Experience.*[b]

As his work progressed, the Abbé became convinced that the signs the deaf made with their hands in trying to communicate with each other were the basis of a mother tongue for them, in much the same way that one's native language is for a hearing person. He set himself to expand and elaborate these signs, in order to develop them into a full language, capable of expressing abstract thought, as well as concrete ideas in pantomime. He did not condemn the efforts of others in teaching articulation, but since, in his opinion, the deaf were capable of thought and reason only in the use of signs, he could see no purpose for speech. To him, even writing was, for the deaf, a translation from the sign language. (44,b, p. 42)

De l'Épée recognized the crudeness and inadequacy of the signs developed naturally among the deaf, even though he believed these to be a language native to them. He decided, therefore, to write a dictionary and grammar of signs, refining and organizing them until they became an adequate means of expression.

At first he was appalled at the magnitude of the task. Then he recalled that "the most learned of us ignore more than three thousand words in our language." He decided to ignore many more in the language of signs, as being not necessary in the everyday life of

[a] Instruction of Deaf and Dumb by means of Methodical Signs.
[b] The True Manner of Instructing the Deaf and Dumb, Confirmed by a Long Experience.

the deaf. Any objects near at hand, such as parts of the body, clothing, etc., he would not name in signs. It was enough to point to them. He would not name birds, beasts, tools with which one worked, and such things. A descriptive, pantomimic gesture was sufficient for these. He was more concerned in establishing a means of expression for the ideas not so easily pantomimed.

La Véritable Manière was an elaborate and detailed piece of work. It was planned, not for the use of the deaf themselves, but as a guide for their teachers.

De l'Épée began by stating optimistically that

> the instruction of the deaf and dumb is not at all as difficult as one would ordinarily suppose. It is concerned only with making to enter through their eyes into their mind what would ordinarily enter ours through the ears. (44,b, p. 1)

According to his own account, the Abbé began his instruction of the deaf by teaching them a manual alphabet. A simple word, such as "door," was then written on the blackboard in large letters, while the pupils spelled out the letters on their fingers. They were then shown the door of the classroom, and taught to write the word. In this way, he said, his pupils learned as many as twenty-four words in three days' time.

Verbs were taught by dramatizing the action and spelling out the word. In an early lesson described by de l'Épée, the sentence to be taught was, "I carry." To make clear the meaning of the pronoun, he would call a student to stand beside him. With the index finger of the left hand, he pointed to the word "I" written on the blackboard, while he tapped himself on the chest with the right. Then he moved his left forefinger to the word "carry." Taking a large book, he walked about the room, carrying the book under his arm, on his shoulder, on his head, on his back, in a fold of his robe. Returning to the table, he had the student repeat the same actions, while the teacher pointed to the word "you" on the blackboard and also to the student, being careful to look at the student rather than the class, to illustrate the second person pronoun. (44,b, pp. 6-7)

Other pronouns and verbs were taught in similar fashion. De l'Épée explained constantly that every presentation of language must be such that the pupils could understand and use it, in order to develop their intelligence.

For the articles, de l'Épée invented brief signs. He showed his pupils the joints of his fingers, and indicated that the small words used as articles joined other words in the same way that our joints joined our bones. (To the grammarians, he extended a parenthetical apology for the inaccuracy of the definition.) A finger crooked at the joint was, therefore, the sign of an article. Carried to the head to touch a hat, it was masculine, and to the ear at the edge of the feminine headdress, it was feminine.

In this fashion, de l'Épée went down through the grammar of the French language, inventing some sort of gesture which he applied to each element and used to teach language to his deaf pupils. As their language became more involved, he combined signs in one expression to indicate the various elements of a thought.

He was very meticulous in his explanations for abstract ideas. His definition of "I believe" was a typical example:

I believe
- I think *yes* (pointing to forehead and making sign *yes*)
- I say *yes* with my heart (pointing to heart and making sign *yes*)
- I say *yes* with my mouth (pointing to mouth and making sign *yes*)
- I do not see with my eyes (pointing to eyes and making sign *no*) (41,b, p. 129)

Each verb was accompanied by signs for its mood and tense, each noun by signs for number and gender, in addition to the basic gesture, which was a mimetic representation of the action or object. Although the four or five signs needed to express a word in this fashion were made, "in the twinkling of an eye," they were still too long and involved for ordinary conversation. The Abbé, therefore, shortened them to mere indications of the original signs. He called these "signes raccourcis" or shortened signs. (8,b, p. 47) The normal abbreviations that would develop in daily use no doubt helped the shortening process.

The second section of the book was a description of the techniques used in teaching the deaf to speak. First, de l'Épée gave warm and unstinting praise to Amman and Bonet for their work with the deaf. Their books he called "two flames" which made clear his way to teaching articulation.

Then he described his own methods, which he considered an

improvement, in "trying to teach a deaf-mute to pronounce a word." First, he "began by having him wash his hands until they were very clear." Then he traced an *a* on the table and, taking his pupil's hand, placed the fourth finger in his mouth up to the second knuckle, and pronounced the vowel strongly, calling the student's attention to the position of the tongue. In this way he went through each speech position, having the student imitate him, placing his finger in his own mouth and pronouncing the sound in the same way. He thought of an ingenious method to illustrate the trill of the French sound for *r* by placing water in his mouth and gargling it.

From single elements, he went on to drill his pupils in practicing the pronounciation of syllables, until they finally reached the articulation of simple words. Lipreading was a natural corollary to articulation, since the pupils, in imitating the teacher's speech movements, also learned at the same time to understand them.

In the end, de l'Épée decided that articulation and lipreading, while entirely possible, were not worth the time and effort necessary to teach them to the deaf. He made a point of the fact that the "lip alphabet," as he called it, was different in each language, while the manual alphabet and signs could be applied to all languages. Since he was still of the opinion that the deaf could think only in signs and gestures, he saw little reason to make the effort to teach them what he felt was for them an artificial language. (44,b)

De l'Épée's establishment was not only a school, but a home for his pupils. There he lived with them, attending to their physical needs, supplying food, clothing, and shelter as well as education. The place was soon known as a refuge for any deaf-mute in need of help.

The story was told of a young deaf-mute boy, lost and ragged, found wandering alone in the streets of Paris. He was brought to the school of de l'Épée where he was warmly received. Since he could give himself no name, the Abbé called him Theodore, the gift of God.

As time went on, and the boy's education progressed, de l'Épée was more and more convinced that he came from a wealthy family. He was bright and quick to learn. As he became able to express himself, he described things he remembered in his former life that indicated a home of wealth and culture. He told how he was brought to the city in fine clothes, which were taken from him in exchange for rags, when he was sent out to wander by himself. But still he had no words for his family name nor his home city.

When he was grown to manhood, de l'Épée sent him out with another student and a hearing teacher from the school to tour

France and see if they could discover his origin. For months they traveled through the cities of France with no success. As they were about to give up the quest and return to Paris, they came to the outskirts of Toulouse. Theodore gave excited indications of recognition. They entered the city, and before the gates of the Count of Solar he stopped and pointed out his home.

Discreet inquiries were made concerning the family of the count. It was learned that the son and heir of the family was a deaf-mute who had, it was said, died in Paris years before. A cousin had inherited and now held the title and estates.

The Abbé de l'Épée, convinced that his young pupil was the rightful heir, fought his cause so vigorously in the courts that a judgment was brought in his favor and the heritage awarded to young Theodore. But the wheels of justice turned so slowly that, before the decree was carried out, the old Abbé died. The cousin who held the inheritance immediately declared Theodore an impostor and appealed to have the decision reversed. Without the support of his protector, Theodore lost his case. In despair, he joined a regiment of cuirassiers in active service, threw himself into the forefront of the fighting, and was killed in his first battle. (168,a)

In 1788, the Abbé de l'Épée, then an old man, finding his funds for the school running low, had denied himself fuel in his own rooms in the bitter cold of winter, to save money. His pupils and friends begged him to use some warmth for the sake of his health. He yielded to their entreaty, but with a deep sense of guilt, and lamented at how much he robbed his "children" by this self-indulgence.

He died on December 23, 1789, at the age of 77, beloved of his pupils and the teachers he had trained, and famous in all of Europe for his work with deaf-mutes. (91)

Upon the death of the Abbé de l'Épée, a successor was needed to take his place, and a commission of the Academy of Science was appointed to choose a permanent successor. In the interim, the school was directed by M. Alloy, according to one authority. (91, p.14) Another report indicated that this position was held by the Abbé Masse. (168,a)

In Bordeaux, in the south of France, was one of the men who had trained as a teacher of the deaf under de l'Épée. This man was Roch Ambroise Cucurron Sicard, born September 23, 1742, at Fosseret. (91, p. 59) When the Archbishop of Bordeaux, Monseigneur de Cicé, attracted by the work of de l'Épée, had decided to open a school for the deaf in his own diocese, he chose Sicard, a young priest in his district, to go to Paris for training. De l'Épée found him particularly suited for the work, and often commented favorably on his skill in teaching. Sicard opened the school at Bordeaux in 1782, and was very successful.

At the death of de l'Épée, there were four candidates for the position of director of the school in Paris, all of whom had been trained by de l'Épée. From these four, the commission selected Sicard. In 1790, Louis XVI ratified the appointment. In that same year, the school was moved to the Celestine Convent, which had been declared state property by the National Assembly, and was given a government grant for the support of the work. At this time, the school for the blind was associated in the same establishment with the school for the deaf. (91)

In the autumn of 1792, Sicard was caught in the frenzy of the September Massacres of the French Revolution, and very nearly lost his life.

On August 26, a municipal officer and sixty armed men entered the Institute for the Deaf and Dumb and arrested Sicard as a non-conforming priest. He was imprisoned for the night, with many more, in the large hall of a hotel.

At his school, the dismay and consternation of his pupils and teachers was promptly organized into action. Led by Massieu, one of the most capable of the deaf, they wrote a petition, which they succeeded in presenting to the National Assembly the next morning.

> Mr. President:
>   They have taken from the deaf and dumb their fosterer, their guardian, and their father. They have shut him up in prison as if he were a thief and a murderer. But he has not killed, he has not stolen. He is not a bad citizen. His whole time is spent in teaching us to love virtue and our country. He is good, just, and pure. We ask of you his liberty. Restore him to his children, for we are his children. He loves us as if he were our father. It is he who has taught us all we know. Without him we should be like beasts. Since he was taken away, we have been full of sorrow and distress. Return him to us and you will make us happy. (81, p.72)

The reading of the petition was greeted with applause. Orders were sent to examine the reasons for Sicard's arrest. But in the general confusion the orders were lost and he remained imprisoned.

On the afternoon of September second, the prisoners were forced into the courtyard of the hotel. Twenty-four of them were placed into six carriages for transportation to the prison of the Abbaye. The drivers were ordered to drive slowly, that the prisoners might be massacred by angry mobs along the way.

Sicard was in the first carriage. As they reached the court of the Abbaye, the frightened prisoners leaped from the carriage, to be killed one by one as they did so. The fourth man escaped into the building, although covered with sabre wounds. Thinking the first carriage empty, the mob turned their attention to the second one, and Sicard made his escape into the building, unnoticed.

He reached the Hall of the Committee, and begged for their protection. This they promised, as soon as they knew who he was. As he stood among the men of the Committee, some from the mob recognized him, and one came with a pike to thrust him through. Monnet,[a] a watchmaker, interposed his body between the weapon's point and Sicard, saying,

> It is the Abbé Sicard, one of the most useful men in the country and father of the deaf and dumb. Your weapons shall pass through my body before they reach him.

The mob drew back, and Sicard leaped into an open window to repeat his plea to the whole crowd. The crowd answered,

> We must spare Sicard. He is too valuable a man to die. His whole life is filled with benevolent labors. He has no time to be a conspirator.

They seized him and tried to carry him triumphantly to freedom. But he insisted that his liberty must come through legal channels. So they left him with the Committee, which did not know what to do with him. When he begged for a place to sleep, they put him in a small adjoining room, with two other prisoners.

All night, the Committee calmly continued its business, while the frenzied mob carried on their questioning and massacre of priests in the court under the windows. Sicard and his two companions stood at their window and watched and listened.

When all the priests in the court had been killed, the crowd decided to find Sicard and kill him. They began battering at the outer door of the small room. To the pleas of the prisoners at the inner door, begging to be let out of their now dangerous sanctuary, the Committee coolly answered that they had lost the key. The prisoners saw a loft over their heads. Sicard's companions decided that if one of them could be saved, he was the one most needed. With much persuasion, they finally induced him to climb on their shoulders, and so reach the loft and hide there. But before the outer

[a] Variously spelled, Monot, Monnot, and Monet.

door gave way, two more priests were dragged into the court and the crowd turned to them and forgot Sicard. So he climbed down again.

The massacres in the court continued for another twenty-four hours. Then some new prisoners brought word that the assassins had retired, saying they would come back for Sicard at four o'clock. Sicard sent a letter to a friend in the Assembly, describing his peril. The Assembly ordered his release, but the order never came through. Then Sicard sent three more notes to influential friends. The third of these went to a lady whose two deaf daughters Sicard had taught. The lady was not at home, but one of the daughters ran with the note to an official who was influential enough to secure Sicard's release.

Fortunately, a tempest of rain delayed the return of the assassins. It was not until seven o'clock that Monnet, the watchmaker, and another member of the Assembly finally managed to release Sicard. (81; 168,b)

He went immediately to his apartment to remove the seals placed upon his doors, and to show himself, safe and well, to his distracted pupils. He was advised not to remain at home yet, for fear the angry mob might return and seize him again. So he went some distance away to the home of Lacombe, who sheltered him. There he was visited by his devoted pupil, Massieu. (81)

There are conflicting reports on what happened to Sicard during the next few years. One authority stated that Sicard was "arrested August 26, 1792, and did not re-enter the Institution until 1796." (43,b, p. 83) During his absence, Alloy again acted as chief of the establishment. In his capacity, he presented a petition to the legislative body for support to assure the continuation of the present schools and the creation of others. The Council passed a tax of fifty centimes, to be levied on the birth of every child, and used to support the schools for deaf-mute and blind. (91, pp. 14-15)

Another authority remarked that, "alas the history of the misfortune of this beneficial man" did not end with his release from the massacres, since for two years more he was outlawed and wandering, "while one invoked in vain the pity that was stirred for him in the hearts of the assassins." (81, p. 290) Another author stated that Sicard fled from Paris and did not see his pupils again for two years, while Degérando took his place at the school. (43,b, p. 83)

During his exile, he took refuge in the suburbs of Saint-Morceau, and used his leisure to compose his *Grammaire Generale* and the *Cours d'Instruction*. (91, p. 59)

The most ambitious of Sicard's writings, *Théorie des Signes* (Theory of Signs) was an elaborate dictionary of signs. In the preface of this book, Sicard eulogized the work of de l'Épée and declared himself dedicated to expanding and carrying on what his predecessor had begun. (120,b)

The work was in two volumes. The first volume was devoted to words that are necessary "for all the physical qualities and functions of man." It was made up mostly of nouns, and of adjectives descriptive of concrete things. The actions of men, intellectual and moral, and the signs for the parts of grammar formed the second volume. Sicard followed de l'Épée's principle of limiting his arbitrary signs to words for which a pantomimic gesture would not suffice.

The words in Sicard's dictionary were arranged, not alphabetically, but according to classes of general ideas. Each group of words was described by a system of signs, all based on the mimetic sign for the original root word. Thus, the descriptive gesture for "house" formed the root sign, with additions, for such words as hamlet, village, city, castle, palace, church, hotel, etc.

The series of signs described to express an idea were soon abbreviated in practical use to a gesture shorthand that had little obvious relationship to the original form. In Volume II of the *Théorie des Signes,* Sicard defined the word "presser" (to urge) in this fashion:

> Presser (to urge): Sign 1—Represent two people, one of whom is working slowly and indifferently.
>
> Sign 2—Represent the other person, urging the first one to be more diligent, to hurry, to move with more speed and vivacity.
>
> Sign 3—Sign of the indefinite mood. (120, b, p. 347)

According to Arnold, these signs were abbreviated to the point that urgently striking the left elbow with the right forefinger was sufficient to indicate the verb "to urge." (8,b, p. 49)

At the end of the book, there was a chart of a manual alphabet, with pictures of the positions of the fingers shaping each letter of the alphabet. It was essentially the same as the one pictured in Bonet's book, published two centuries earlier, which is still in almost universal use among the deaf, wherever manual spelling is taught and used.

The book closed with an account of the life of Jean Massieu, called *Notice sur L'Enfance de Massieu, Sourd-Muet de Naissance, Élève de M. L'Abbé Sicard.*[a]

There has been some question among authorities concerning the teachers in Massieu's life. Saint-Sernin of Bordeaux has been named as his first teacher, and the one who gave him his basic understanding of language. (60)

Massieu's own account, as quoted by Sicard, told the following tale:

Jean Massieu was one of a family of six children, three boys and three girls, all deaf-mutes. Until he was thirteen years and nine months old, Jean remained at home, without instruction. He communicated by means of gestures with his parents and his brothers and sisters, but complained bitterly that strangers could not understand him.

When he saw other children going to school and learning to read and write, he went to his father with a book in his hands, showed him that he could not read it, and demanded to be sent to school, like other children, to learn to read. His father tried to make him understand that he could not go to school because he was deaf.

"At that I cried very hard."[b] He put his fingers into his ears and demanded that his father cure them. Again his father tried to explain that he could not.

Without telling his parents, the boy slipped out of the house and went to school. There he presented himself to the teacher and demanded by gestures to be taught to read and write. The teacher refused him harshly and drove him away from the school. This made him weep again. At home, he tried desperately to trace the shapes of letters with a pen, but they told him nothing.

One day a neighbor, M. de Puymorin, was attracted by the boy. He took him to his house and gave him food and drink. What he observed must have pleased him, for when he went to Bordeaux soon after, he spoke of him to Sicard, who was teaching the school for deaf at Bordeaux at that time. Sicard wrote to Jean's father and offered to educate his promising young son. The letter was explained to Jean. The neighbors thought he was going away to be taught the cooper's trade, but his father told him he was to learn to read and write.

So he traveled with his father to Bordeaux, where he met M. l'Abbé Sicard for the first time. " I found him very skinny," said the boy, naively. He stayed with Bordeaux for three and a half years,

---

[a] An Account of the Childhood of Massieu, Deaf-Mute from Birth, Pupil of M. l'Abbé Sicard.

[b] Alors je criai trés-haut.

and then transferred with Sicard when he was sent to the school at Paris.

According to Sicard, it had always been his impression, and that of his teachers, that the mind of a deaf person was blank, like a white page that has not yet been written upon. He was much interested in asking his pupils, after they had acquired some skill in communication, what they had thought before they came to school.

Massieu was asked what he had thought when, as a child, he saw people looking at each other and moving their lips. He replied that he thought they were expressing ideas. In explanation, he told how someone, who had seen him in mischief, went and spoke to his father. At once, his father came and threatened him with punishment. Also, a relative living in the house used to tell him that he "saw with his ears" a person not yet in sight. Immediately afterward the person would appear.

Massieu's teachers were amazed at the sense and clarity of his ideas before he had any teaching. Sicard confessed that he found his previous concern over a deaf-mute's lack of understanding quite out of proportion to the fact, and rather unnecessary, after he learned from them how much thought and imagination they were capable of on their own account. (120,b)

By the time of Sicard's death, in 1822, the "silent method" of teaching the deaf by signs rather than by speech had come to be known as the French method. The system was first built up in the school of de l'Épée and carried on, along with finger spelling and writing, by Sicard and Saint-Sernin.

Sicard's successor at the school in Paris was Roch Ambroise Auguste Bébian, born August 4, 1789 at Point-à-Pitre, Guadeloupe. He was sent to France for his education, under Sicard. He also taught at the Paris Institute while it was under the direction of Sicard, attaching to himself, as assistant, the young deaf pupil, Laurent Clerc.

By this time the methodical signs had proved too unwieldy to be practical and were breaking down. Both Sicard and Bébian realized, more than did de l'Épée, the very real need of the deaf for a functional use of the language of the people around them. So the school of Bébian reverted, first to "natural" gestures and the manual alphabet, which was then translated into written French. Even this route to the use of language soon seemed too round-about for Bébian.

In 1817, he published his *Essai sur les Sourds-Muets et sur*

Langage Naturel.[a] In 1822, after the death of Sicard, he revised *Manuel d'Enseignement Pratique des Sourds-Muets,*[b] which was then adopted by the Council of the Administration. Because of the discord of opinions concerning the fundamental methods of teaching the handicapped, Bébian determined to provoke an independent discussion, and created the Journal of Instruction for Deaf-Mute and Blind. He published his booklet, *Lecture Instantanée,* or Methods of Teaching Reading without Spelling (i.e., finger spelling). He reprinted *L'Education de Sourd-Muets,* "placing at the door of their first teachers and all parents a new method of learning language without translation," (i.e., without translation from manual signs). (91, p. 66)

In order to have more freedom to carry out his own ideas, he left the Paris Institute and, refusing offers from Saint Petersburg and New York, founded his own school on the boulevard of Montparnasse in Paris. Lack of funds kept him from continuing this venture. In 1832, at the death of l'Abbé Huey, director of the school at Rouen, he was offered that position by the Mayor of Rouen, at the recommendation of the Minister of the Interior. He remained as director of the school at Rouen until 1834, when ill health forced him to resign.

He left France, going back to Pointe-à-Pitre with his wife and son, where he died, February 24, 1839.

An earlier contemporary of these teachers, one Ernaud, was also working with deaf pupils, along much the same lines as those developed by Pereira. Ernaud was particularly interested in stimulating any residual hearing his pupils might have, and claimed much success in developing that sense by means of a series of graduated auditory training exercises, "for those not entirely deprived." One stimulation he used was to place a cornet against a pupil's ear and sound it.

He stated that he had known only one case of total deafness. When he found it impossible to re-animate any hearing in a pupil, he taught him lipreading and speech by visual means.

In 1757, he demonstrated two of his deaf boys before the Academy of Science. He had taught them to lipread, and to identify invisible speech sounds by touching the throat of the speaker. (42, Vol. I, p. 431; 72, p. 324)

Ernaud felt that sign language was not comparable to a mother tongue for the deaf, since it was a form of communication they

[a] Essay on the Deaf Mutes and Natural Language.
[b] Manual of Practical Instruction for Deaf-Mutes.

invented themselves which was at variance with the language around them. However, he admitted using sign language himself, for necessary explanations to his pupils, before they knew any other language.

He thought Russian, Polish, and English were the languages most easily learned by the deaf-mute, the first two because of being free of articles, and the last because of its simplicity of syntax. Those which he learned with the most difficulty, according to Ernaud, were Spanish, Portuguese, French, but above all, German. (42, Vol. II, pp. 24-25)

Pereira attacked Ernaud bitterly, calling him a copyist and re-asserting his own claim as the inventor of the art of teaching language to deaf pupils. It was difficult to substantiate Pereira's claim of plagiarism, since he refused to divulge his method for comparison, but it seemed evident that the two men were following somewhat different methods, the one depending entirely upon speech, and the other employing also a form of dactylology.

In any case, the Academy encouraged Ernaud, although they felt the pupils he exhibited were not as far advanced as those of Pereira. (42, Vol. I, pp. 430-434)

Of the same period in France, was another priest, Claude Francis Deschamps, who also devoted his life to teaching the deaf. He was a pupil of Amman, and was convinced of the value of speech and lipreading for his deaf pupils. He tried for a time to work with de l'Épée. But he could not bring himself to continue in a method in which he did not believe. So he withdrew from Paris and opened a small private school in Orleans. Here he taught speech and lipreading, together with reading and writing, because he felt they aided each other. He used flash cards to build words, and a manual alphabet for dictation, in order to multiply and vary the exercises. He even taught his pupils to read letters in raised relief and to lipread by touch, so that they could communicate in the darkness of the night. When he felt they were needed, he used mimetic signs. His first object was to teach religion, and "God" was the first word he presented to his deaf pupils.

He took paying pupils, when they came to him, but he also took the poor free of charge, and supported the school, as much as was necessary, from his own income.

In 1779, he published a book entitled *Cours Elementaire d'Education des Sourds-Muets*.[a] The Royal Society of Medicine

---

[a] An Elementary Course in the Education of Deaf-Mutes.

examined his work and gave him their approval. (42, Vol. I, pp. 441-445)

It has also been stated that he was equally zealous in his efforts in behalf of those born blind. Said one authority,

> He is the first in France, if we are not mistaken, who has outlined the features of the art which teaches the latter reading and writing.[a]

Joseph-Marie Degérando[b] was born at Lyon, France, February 22, 1772, the son of an architect. As a young man, he joined the army of the young Lyonnaise rebels, and later exiled himself in Switzerland. After the amnesty, he returned to his family, and was married to Annette Rathsanhausen in December, 1799. (91, p. 63)

The Baron Degérando was a statesman and a philanthropist, who was interested in the problems of language, and was led to a study of the langugage problems of the deaf. The Council for the Administration of the Royal Institution for Deaf-Mutes set him the task of compiling and evaluating the various methods used in teaching deaf-mutes, in various countries, both in the past and up to his own time. He expressed himself as intimated by the tremendous task, when he began to study the vast contradictions, controversies, and animosities he found in the literature. He "searched in vain for an impartial arbiter," and finally decided to present the facts as he found them as impartially as he could, simply to report and not to judge. (34)

The result was his magnificent two-volume history, *De l'Education des Sourds-Muets de Naissance,*[c] published in 1827. In this book he covered, in a most thorough manner, the history of the education of the deaf from the earliest records to his own day. He set the various methods against each other, comparing and analyzing advantages and disadvantages in each. He did not neglect the personalities of the men who were the key figures in the history, but his chief emphasis was on a description and evaluation of their techniques and philosophies. (42)

Degérando became president of the Council of the Administration of the Royal Institution for Deaf-Mutes and, in this capacity, was presented, on April 24, 1840, with a bust of the Abbé de l'Épée. (91, p. 40)

---

[a] Il est premier, en France, si nous ne nous trompons, qui ait tracé les lineaments de l'art qui enseigne à ceux-ci la lecture et l'écriture. (42, Vol. I, p. 445))
[b] Also frequently spelled de Gérando.
[c] Of the Education of Those Deaf-Mute from Birth.

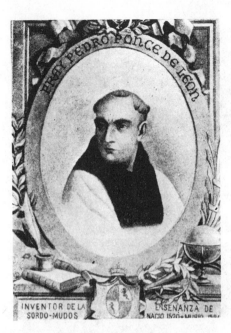

PLATE I. Pedro de Ponce de Leon, "Inventor of the Teaching of Deaf and Dumb. Born 1520—Died 1584." From *Il Metodo Orale al Lume delle più Moderne Acquisizioni Scientifiche,* by P. Giovanni Bonuccelli, 1956.

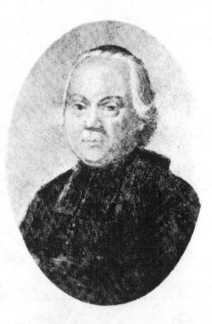

PLATE II. Charles Michel de l'Épée. From *De Eerste Eeuw van het Instituut voor Doofstommen te Groningen,* by J. G. Brugmans, 1896.

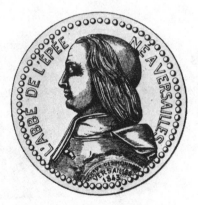

PLATE III. L'Abbé de l'Épée—Medallion. From *Etude Bibliographique et Iconographique sur l'Abbé de l'Épée,* by Aldolphe Belanger, 1886.

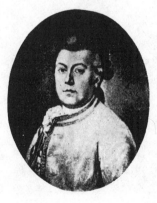

PLATE IV. Samuel Heinicke. From *Samuel Heinicke Gesammelte Schriften,* by Georg and Paul Schumann, 1912.

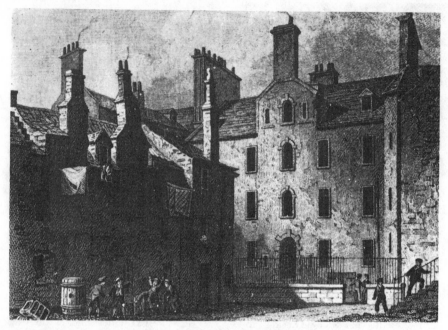

PLATE V. School for the Deaf and Dumb, Edinburgh, 1819. From an uncopyrighted photograph in the Edinburgh Library.

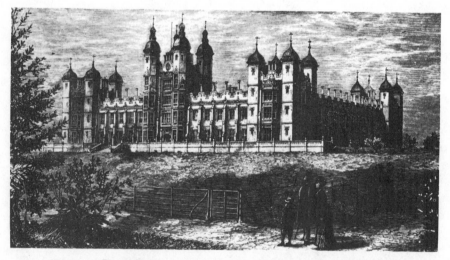

PLATE VI. Donaldson's Hospital, School for Deaf and Dumb, Edinburgh, 1850. From an uncopyrighted photograph in the Edinburgh Library.

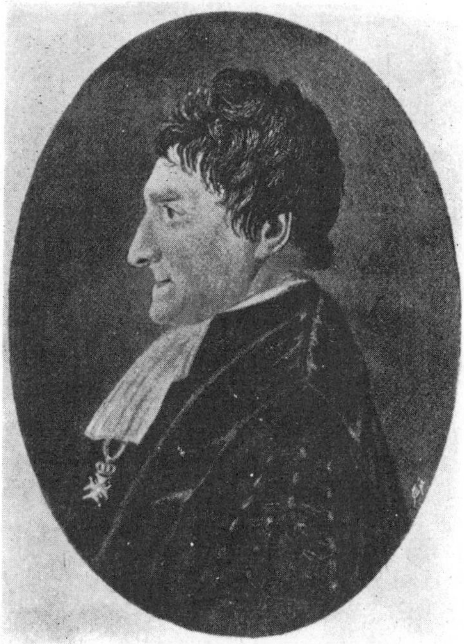

PLATE VII. Henry Daniel Guyot. From *Eerste Eeuw van het Instituut voor Doofstomme te Groningen,* by J. G. Brugmans, 1896.

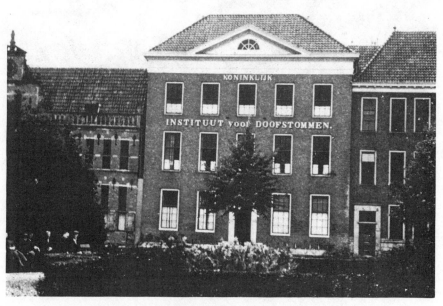

PLATE VIII. Institution for the Deaf and Dumb, Groningen. From a photograph by the author.

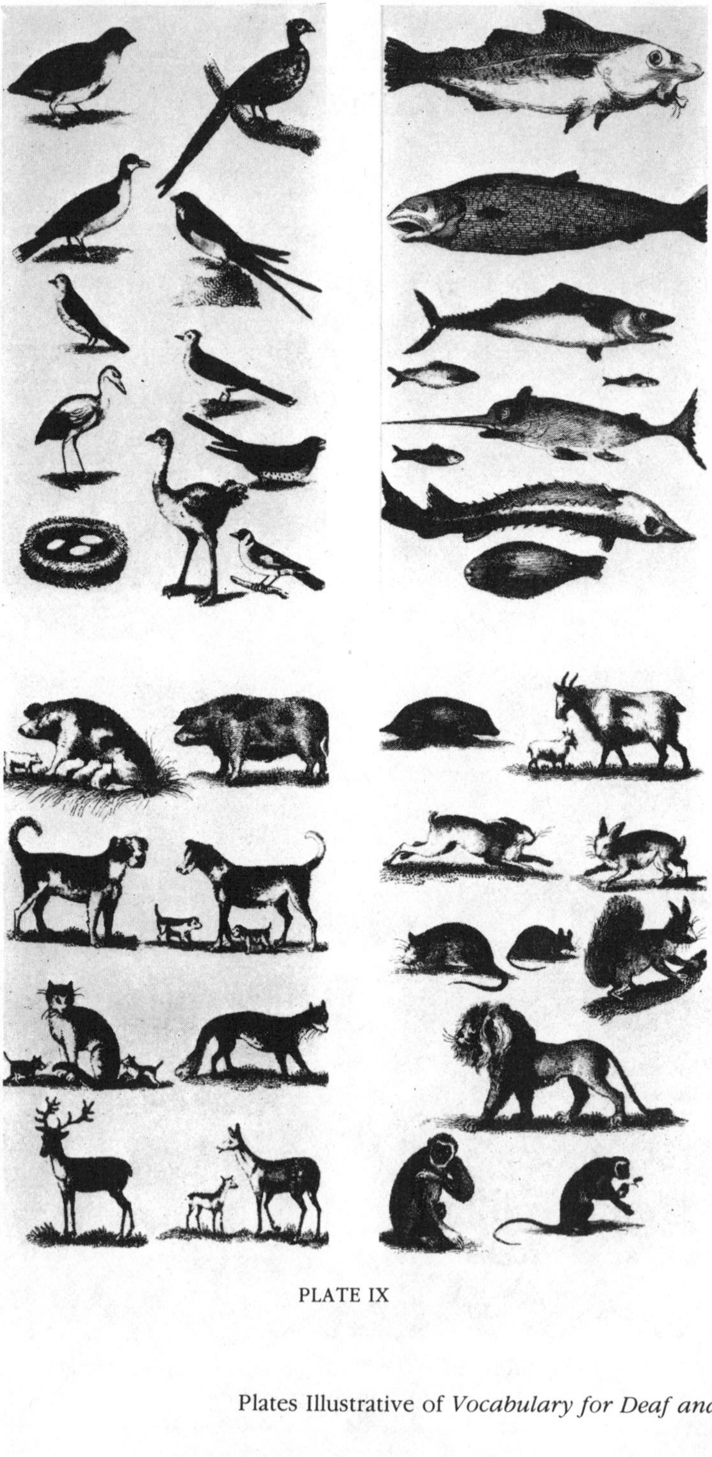

PLATE IX

Plates Illustrative of *Vocabulary for Deaf and Dumb.*

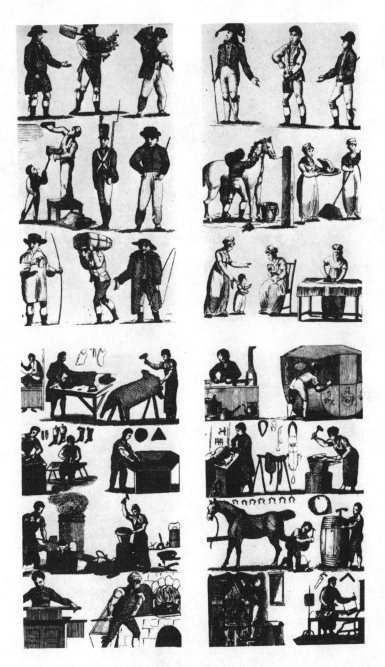

PLATE X

From the book of the same title, by Joseph Watson, 1810.

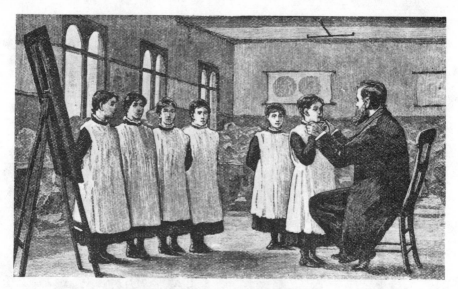

PLATE XI. Teaching the Dumb to Speak—Richard Elliott and Pupils. From
Deaf-and-Dumb Land, by Joseph Hatton.

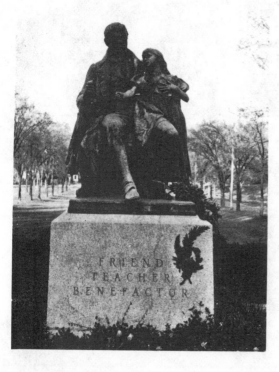

PLATE XII. Thomas Hopkins
Gallaudet and Alice Cogswell.
Permission of Edmund
Boatner, Superintendent
American School for the Deaf,
Hartford, Connecticut, 1959.

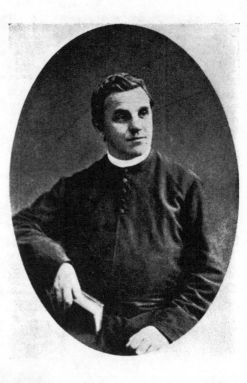

PLATE XIII. Guilio Tarra. From *Il Metodo Orale al Lume delle più Moderne Acquisizioni Scientifiche,* by P. Giovanni Bonnuccelli, 1956.

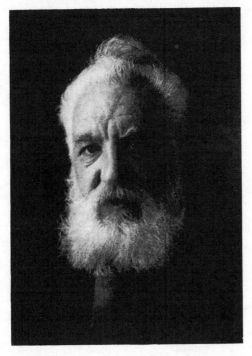

PLATE XIV. Alexander Graham Bell. By permission of The Volta Bureau.

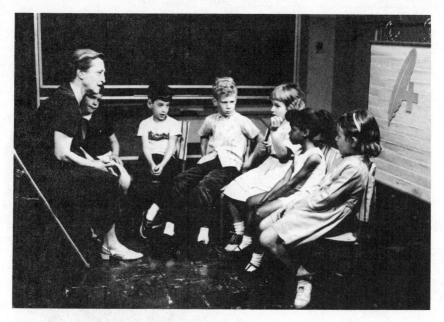

PLATE XV. Dr. Bender teaching a language class at the Cleveland Hearing and Speech Center. Photo, courtesy United Appeal.

SPAIN

Lorenzo Hervas y Panduro (1735-1809), a celebrated Spanish philologist, was first a professor of philosophy at Madrid, then a Jesuit missionary in America. When the Jesuits were proscribed in America, he went to Italy. Here he served as Prefect of the Quirinal Library in Rome, for a time, before returning to Madrid.

The available literature is not clear on the reasons for his keen interest in the deaf. His contribution to the field was a book published in Madrid in 1795. It was called *Escuela Española de Sordo-Mudos, o Arte Para Enseñarles a Escribir y Hablar el Idioma Español.*[a] The book was an unusually comprehensive and scholarly piece of work. Published in two volumes, it covered the whole field of language for the deaf, in Spanish, both manual and oral. There was a section on Portuguese as well, but in less detail, since parallels could be drawn from the previous discussion of Spanish. Another section related a comprehensive account of the history of the deaf and earlier efforts at their education.

In the introduction, Hervas commented that those who read in his book the techniques for teaching writing and speech to deaf-mutes would believe such work to be more difficult than it was in actual practice. The teaching of arts and sciences, he added, was also difficult, and required even more effort from the learner than from the teacher. Why should not the teacher, then, exert himself, cheerfully, to pass on to others what he had himself once been taught with equal effort. (72, Vol. I, p. IV)

In discussing the deaf and dumb, Hervas considered that, of the two afflictions, deafness was by far the more important, because, he said, it was not only the cause of the muteness, but also prevented the deaf person from understanding what others said to him.

He went on to say that the instruction of the deaf-mute was advantageous not only to himself but to the whole of society, since it restored him to his proper place among his fellows. The deaf-mute, being accustomed to his condition, was not always aware of the extent of his misfortune. This did not lessen the responsibility of his teachers, since the Creator meant all men to live rationally with their brothers, and to earn all the bounty for which God has enriched their senses.

The second chapter described the causes of deafness, and of muteness among the deaf. Hervas stated, without question, that the

---

[a] Spanish School for Deaf-Mutes or Art of Teaching them to Write and Speak the Spanish Language.

deaf-mute were mute through no defect of the vocal organs, which were rarely affected, but only because through lack of hearing they could hear neither their own voices, to regulate them, nor the voices of others, to imitate them. (72, pp. 3-22)

The succeeding chapters covered in great detail the positions of the speech organs for the utterance of each speech sound, with graded exercises for the combination of elements into syllables. There were careful charts, diagramming the grammatical structure of the Spanish language. Considerable attention was given to lipreading. The author made the comment that,

> It is said in the schools for the deaf that girls are better lipreaders than boys. (72, Vol. I, p. 287)

This early comment is particularly interesting in the light of our modern findings that with normal children language and speech emerge earlier and more readily among girls than among boys.

Hervas had the idea that a young child could more easily learn such a skill than an older one. He tried it for a series of lessons with a little deaf boy of twenty-seven months. The baby learned much more readily than an adult, who was also a deaf-mute. (72, Vol. I, p. 289)

Apparently the experiment ended with this one case.

The book contained an excellent chart of a manual alphabet similar to Bonet's. In teaching new vocabulary in writing, Hervas advocated using the manual letters to indicate the parts of speech, V to be associated with verbs and N with nouns. (72, Vol II, p. 14)

Hervas also discussed the work of de l'Épée and his language of signs with a great deal of approval. He included quite an extensive dictionary of signs for Spanish schools, describing the gestures used to define words in much the same way as did de l'Épée.

He once visited, he said, a certain Baltasar Caracioli, who was interested in the ancient pantomime language of Greek drama. The two of them decided to see if a deaf-mute could more readily understand gesture language than a hearing person. They chose a deaf-mute boy of ten, and took him through a series of shops of various kinds, teaching him to describe by gesture the things he saw. The boy did this with a great deal of readiness, learning the pantomime language more quickly than a hearing boy. At times Hervas and Caracioli could not understand a new pantomimic gesture that the boy used, at which he would go back to known signs, and by means of much circumlocution bring them to understand. He invented new signs as he needed them more readily than his guides. (72, Vol. I, p. 281)

This experiment was supposed to support de l'Épée's contention that signs are a natural language for the deaf. After the experimenters had satisfied their own curiosity about it, that seemed to end the matter for them.

One most unusual detail about this book, published in 1795, was the author's constant acknowledgement of other authorities. The lightest reference to another author was invariably accompanied by a footnote giving exactly the title, chapter, and page from which the reference was taken. It is surprising that succeeding authorities have made so little reference to the work of Hervas.

Of the schools for the deaf in Spain at this time, we know very little, aside from the rather oblique references in Hervas to their existence.

ITALY

The opening of the first school in Italy has been credited to the Abba Silvestri. He established a school for deaf in Rome in 1784. He was trained by de l'Épée, but also studied the techniques of Amman and was acquainted with the publications of Hervas. Apparently, he attempted to teach by a combination of these diverse methods and found it a rather ineffective compromise. (44,b, p. 228; 8,b, p. 103; 75, pp. 134-135) It remained for his successor to select one method from among them all and make the school a success.

GERMANY

German schools of the eighteenth century became the champions of the oral method of teaching the deaf. During the second half of the century, Otto Lasius, a pastor in Burgdorff, taught language to deaf pupils by means of reading and writing.

J. F. L. Arnoldi, pastor at Giessen, taught lipreading and speech to his deaf pupils, as well as reading and writing. A Hessian nobleman, who had a deaf son with a particularly bright and personable nature, asked Arnoldi to undertake his education. He did so "with zeal animated by affection." His teaching was so successful that he soon added other deaf pupils to his class. Among them were two Swiss girls, who, he said, learned to speak and lipread remarkably well.

Arnoldi believed in a natural approach to language teaching. He took his pupils for walks in public places and showed them new things, then taught them how to express their experiences in words. He invented games and drills, so that repetition might "engrave on the minds" of his pupils the things he taught them.

He remarked how pleased the deaf were when the words they pronounced were understood by others. Once they developed this skill, he said, they often talked to themselves alone, and even talked in their dreams.

He estimated that four or five years of age was the most fruitful time to begin the education of a deaf child, the younger age being the more favorable for forming the habits of the delicate articulation organs. But development of ideas was more rapid between ten and eleven.

Arnoldi kept a daily journal of his work. In this he noted that the deaf were often irritable and easily aroused to annoyance, because they expected their signs to be as quickly intelligible to us as our own language. He, therefore, advised that one should neglect no means of gaining the confidence and affection of a deaf-mute, in order to be able to reach his intelligence.

He described and published his methods in 1777, in a book called *Praktische Unterweissung Taubstumme Personnen Reden und Schreiben zu Lehren*.[a] He made much use of pictures to recall absent objects, in his teaching of language. He also used dramatization of action for verbs. He accepted mimetic signs provided they were natural gestures invented spontaneously by his pupils, but he taught no conventional signs. Articulation and oral speech were used wherever he thought it practical, but his chief goal was to teach reading, so that his pupils might, as quickly as possible, make use of books. (42, Vol. I, pp. 367-375)

Germany's foremost name in the education of the deaf, and the man who became known as the "father of the German method" was Samuel Heinicke.

He was born April 10, 1727, in Nautschutz, Germany, near Weissenfels, to Samuel and Rosine Thieme Heinicke. (25, p. 356; 109, p. V) His father was a farmer. Young Samuel had considerable musical talent, and also a strong inclination for a professional life, as a teacher or preacher. His father blocked these ambitions with the blunt order, "You shall remain a farmer." (113, p. V)

The break with his home came at about the age of 24, when his father arranged a marriage for him that was not to his liking. Samuel left home and went to Dresden, where, in 1750, he entered military service as a member of the bodyguard of the Elector of Saxony. (76, p. 12; 113, p. V; 137, p. 706; 168, d)

---

[a] Practical Instructions for Teaching Deaf-Mute Persons to Speak and Write.

His efficiency and intelligence in the execution of his military duties left him free time, which he devoted to study. The military chaplain took an interest in helping him. "In the night's still hours" he studied Latin and French, until he became so proficient that he could read classics in both languages. He also studied mathematics and writing, and took on private tutoring in these subjects. (69; 76; 113; 137)

In 1752, his father offered to buy his release from the military services, if he would come home. This offer Heinicke refused.

By 1754, he had so many private pupils that he could afford to think of marriage. He was married in that year to Johanne Elizabeth Kracht. (69, p. 369; 113, p. V)

At about this time, there appeared among Heinicke's pupils a deaf-mute boy. He had never known a deaf-mute before, but this boy, "whose attention and co-operation raised him to a high level" aroused his interest. Learning to write was not difficult for him, and in arithmetic he made such good progess that "his teacher and his parents were heartily glad." (76, p. 12)

Heinicke tried to find a way to teach his pupil to understand oral as well as written communications. He found Amman's *Surdus Loquens,* and Raphel's account of teaching his deaf daughters. Taught by these methods, the boy soon learned to speak, lipread, and write the names of common objects in the room and about the house. (76, p. 13)

Heinicke was so pleased with this work that he wanted to leave military life altogether and devote himself to teaching deaf children. But the outbreak of the Seven Years War recalled him to his military duties. His plea for a discharge was not granted. So "separated from his wife and a beloved child," he entered the army camp at Pirna.

Here the Saxon army was surrounded and captured by the Prussians. On October 17, the guard to which Heinicke was attached was taken prisoner and imprisoned at Dresden.

In spite of being strongly guarded, Heinicke escaped. Dressed as a fiddler, a violin in his hand, his face disfigured with court plaster, with a false beard and hump-backed, he deceived the sentries, and so made his escape.

He fled to Jena, where he was joined by his wife and child. Here he entered the University in 1757, to continue his studies, making his way by giving music lessons. But the recruiting officer of Jena seemed to recognize him. Fearful of being imprisoned as a deserter, he fled again, and came to Hamburg, where he supported himself again by private tutoring.

In 1760, he obtained a post as secretary to Count Schimmelman, recommended by two of his teacher friends and also because of his beautiful handwriting. He was held in high esteem by the whole household, and could have remained in the position, but he wanted an establishment of his own. When there was a vacancy for the position of schoolmaster and cantor in Eppendorf, near Hamburg, he applied and, through the influence of the Count, was granted the position in 1768. Here he remained, living quietly with his family, for ten years. (69, p. 369; 76, p. 14; 137, p. 706)

Again there appeared among Heinicke's pupils a young deaf boy, thirteen years old, the son of a miller. His success with this boy was "so brilliant" that he was soon demonstrating the boy's accomplishments before the educational and religious leaders about him. This publicity quickly brought him more deaf pupils whose families were seeking help for their handicapped children. Scholars and highly-placed public officials expressed their interest in and approval of Heinicke's successful teaching of deaf children.

There was one dissenting voice. Pastor Granau of Eppendorf had asked for the schoolmaster's position for his nephew, but it was granted to Heinicke. Now he cried out against Heinicke's work, declaring it was wrong to try to change the destiny of the deaf, when God had put his mark on them, and so wished them to live in silence.

But Heinicke refused to be drawn into the controversy, and continued to expand his work. He wanted earnestly to make it his life work, and cast about for a means of doing so. Count Schimmelman heard of his desire, and offered to support him for three years at 1000 thalers annually if he would establish his school at Wansbecke, not far from Hamburg. Heinicke felt compelled to refuse this offer. He needed to set his school in a large city, he decided, not only because he would there find more deaf, but also because there they would be surrounded by an abundance of things for which they would need to learn the language for daily use.

In 1775, his wife died. After this Heinicke seemed anxious to leave the vicinity of Eppendorf. In 1778, he accepted an offer to establish his school at Leipzig. Here he was married again, to a widow named Catherine Elizabeth Morin, the sister of one of his deaf pupils. (113, p. V)

The Elector Friedrich August of Saxony agreed to support the new venture, allowing Heinicke to choose his own methods, and granting him an annual allowance of 400 thalers. Pupils who could do so were to pay tuition, but the poor rural children were to be admitted free of charge.

б 5ЧЗб

On April 14, 1778, the school was officially opened, with nine former pupils brought from his school in Eppendorf. (76, p. 15; 113, p. V)

Heinicke enrolled his sixteen-year-old son Rudolph in the University of Leipzig, and a few years later he also entered his fourteen-year-old son, Carl August Dietrich. He made every effort to establish a strong liaison between his own school and the University, both to give his students a place to cross over into a normal educational situation, and also to establish classes for training teachers of the deaf. He also tried to set up a subscription fund for the education of poor deaf children, and so enlist public interest and support.

None of these plans succeeded. His little private school did not become a free public institution, as he hoped, but continued under the patronage of the Elector of Saxony. For twelve years, Heinicke served as its director, and as the leader of his profession in Germany. On the night of April 29-30, 1790, Samuel Heinicke suffered a stroke and died. (69, p. 369; 76, pp. 15-19)

Heinicke's methods were strictly oral. He stated that "spoken language is the hinge upon which everything turns." First, he insisted, the pupil must learn to take in with his eyes the meaning of the speech of another, then, when he understood the thought, he could be taught the various forms and symbols by which language is expressed. This he must do, "with the eyes steadfastly on the lips, not on the eyes as we do." Heinicke was much opposed to presenting written language first. He was convinced that thought came by means of oral language and written language was but a translation of that thought.

He realized the difficulty the deaf had in remembering the sounds which they were taught to speak but could not hear. Searching for some association with these sounds that would assist recall, he developed the idea of using still another sense to substitute for hearing. Along with sight and touch, he decided to make use of taste.

The vowels seemed to be the sounds that were the most troublesome to remember. So he gave his pupils substances to taste that seemed to him related to these vowel sounds. For the vowel A, he used pure water; for E, wormwood; for I, vinegar; for O, sweet water; for U, olive oil. (8, b, p. 54; 114, b, p. 51)

Heinicke stated in one of his early writings that

> When one remembers that for the deaf the eyes must stand for the ears and for speech must be the hand and writing materials, then one can see the way to teach them . . . It is not difficult to teach them oral speech. Since some years, I have taught deaf-born pupils, and now

there are five in my school, one for four years, who has come so far that he knows about God and the world and can express himself in writing about abstract material and read printed books. He was finally confirmed by Pastor Granau in Eppendorf near Hamburg and accepted for communion. (114,b, pp. 5-8)

He also noted that deaf children cry, laugh, and shout normally, so they do have vocal sounds and can be taught to use them properly.

Heinicke made a great point of the fact that a deaf child was mute simply for lack of ability to learn speech through hearing. He cited as evidence of this truth the speech ability of children born blind and the fact that when hearing could be restored to deaf children muteness disappeared. He was particularly distressed concerning the deaf children who were uselessly subjected to operations on their tongues to correct their lack of speech. (203, p. 87)

He described the partially deaf, who could hear loud sounds, and sometimes even learn a few words, but were unable to distinguish certain speech sounds, such as the sibilant and nasal consonants. Without special teaching, he stated, they were as helpless as the totally deaf in learning language.

He was much disturbed over the common practice of beginning a deaf child's language by teaching him letters. No child ever learned his mother tongue first by letters, he contended. Besides, with this method they needed much patient holding up of mirrors, pressing of tongues and throats, breathing exercises, and finger alphabets. In the end, they tear down with one hand what they build with the other, he said.

Heinicke advocated first teaching words, with functional meaning. Then the words were to be taken apart, into syllables, and finally letters, rather than teaching letters as meaningless hieroglyphics. (67, a, pp. 37-50)

Never accustomed to curbing his temper, Heinicke's forceful nature and vigorous defense of his methods left him few friends and made many enemies. When he heard that the Emperor Joseph had sent the Abbé Stork from Vienna to the school of de l'Épée in Paris, to learn the manual method of teaching the deaf, Heinicke wrote to Stork, telling him that the French method was harmful to educational progress and urging him strongly to adopt instead his own method of oral instruction. Stork was loyally indignant at what seemed to him an unwarranted attack on de l'Épée. He did visit Heinicke's school but felt that Heinicke had exaggerated the benefits of his method, and that the results did not bear out his claims. He remained convinced that the methods he learned in Paris were superior. (71,a, p. 155; 137, p. 369)

De l'Épée at once wrote to Heinicke, in French, defending his own methods and asking questions of Heinicke. When he received an answer from Heinicke, the letter was written "in small German letters, " and did not touch on any of the points that de l'Épée had set out in his letter. De l'Épée then concluded that Heinicke did not know French, as he, himself, did not know German. He wrote again, this time in Latin, a language common to both men. Heinicke replied, although more briefly. The two men exchanged a number of letters, each one describing and defending his own philosophy and techniques, without in the least convincing the other. (44, b, Appendix)

Finally, de l'Épée presented the correspondence to the Zürich Academy,[a] asking that they judge between them and resolve the controversy.

The Academy accepted the task and reviewed the correspondence. They also made an effort to find out more of Heinicke's method, of which they could learn little that was specific because "he refused to divulge it except for money." They expressed themselves as particularly puzzled about his claims to successful results by the use of taste. Concerning the French method they had an abundance of material.

The Academy replied in a letter to de l'Épée, February 6, 1783. They stated that they thought de l'Épée's method was good, because they had seen its results adequately demonstrated. They felt that neither man could claim a method that was "natural," nor exclusively beneficial for teaching the deaf. Of Heinicke's method, they had been able to learn so little that they could not pass judgment. They were inclined to be doubtful of some of his claims, especially after the testimony of the Abbé Stork, who had seen and was not impressed. They stated that, in their judgment, de l'Épée had answered his adversary sufficiently and the controversy could be dropped. (44, a; 71, a)

Heinicke left no direct disciple of his method and pedagogy. Said one biographer, "He was rough and dictatorial in his ways and could not set out his ideas gently, but remained stuck in polemics." (113, p. XII) His son Rudolf died before him, in 1781. Carl and Anton were not interested.

So his widow took over. She was a woman of great intelligence and energy. As assistants, she had a son-in-law, Carl Gottlieb Reich,

---

a The Zürich Academy was a group of scholars, organized to protect and promote the development of science and literature, similar to the Royal Society in England and the Academy of Science in France.

(171, p. 193) and August Friedrich Petschke. (113, pp. X-XI)

Petschke later became the director of the school at Leipzig, and wrote some excellent grammar books, lesson plans, and exercise books for teaching language to deaf children. (100) He advocated forming a community of deaf-mutes, even after their education was completed, where they might live together and earn their living by some sort of manufacturing project, in a sheltered workshop. (42, Vol. I, pp. 34-35)

A young law student, Ernst Adolf Eschke, wandered into Leipzig and became acquainted with the establishment of Samuel Heinicke. He married Heinicke's daughter, and arranged with his father-in-law to dedicate himself to the education of the deaf.

The excellence of the Leipzig Institute made it the inspiration for the opening of others. At the end of 1787, the Prussian Minister, von Zedlitz, suggested to Eschke, then 21, that he come to Berlin to establish a school there. Eschke agreed, but the financial support he expected was not forthcoming. He wrote to the Directors of the College, asking for help. They agreed to sponsor an advertisement in the local papers concerning his work, if it passed their inspection. Pastor Schmidt came to examine his pupils, was well-pleased, and the advertisement was placed in the papers December 2, 1788.

Finding himself still in difficulties, Eschke moved his little school to Nieder-Schönhausen, on the outskirts of Berlin, in 1792, where he remained until 1797. His wife, who was Heinicke's daughter and had his energetic nature, helped with the children, taking care of their board and housekeeping chores. Visitors to the school remarked on the warmth and cheerful understanding between the youngsters and their foster parents. Lessons were given in speech, reading, writing, arithmetic, German composition and letter writing, and the elements of drawing and music, especially singing. Of the latter, they could learn very little, but Eschke tried to give them an idea of music.

But his dream was still a school in Berlin. Gradually he gained more government support, and in March, 1796, he was asked to select a site. He chose a place in Linienstrasse, No. 110, a fine big building with a yard and garden, on the edge of the city. King Friedrich Wilhelm III gave his approval. (134, p. 7)

Now he was able to hire teachers to help him. He published readers, which he used in his own school, trying to improve on the monotonous vocabulary lists that were in common use at the time, and furnished material that would catch the interest of his pupils. These were printed in Latin as well as German letters, so that the pupils could learn to read both. (53)

Eschke died after a short illness, June 17, 1811, at the age of 45. (134, p. 32) His widow received a pension from the profits of the school.

Ludwig Grasshoff, a teacher of Eschke's for two years, took charge of the school, by order of the Directors of the College. Since the teaching of the deaf in northern Germany was a monopoly of the Heinicke family, Grasshoff went to Leipzig to appeal to Reich, the head of the family and school there, for a right to work in Berlin. The Prussian government supported his claim and expanded the school in Berlin.

In November of 1812, there came from the provinces, a young man by the name of Ferdinand Neumann, who applied to Grasshoff for a position as apprentice teacher, to learn the profession. Grasshoff was strongly opposed, saying that he had enough to do to teach the children, without taking time to train new teachers. But this time the Department of Education stepped into the argument, telling Grasshoff that his Institute did not belong to him and he was wrong to try to keep his methods a family secret, but should share them freely, for the good of all. Neumann was accepted, and from then on the Berlin school carried a double responsibility, to train teachers as well as to teach children. (134, p. 33)

Neumann, a young man full of ideas for progress, did not always agree with Grasshoff. He received money for travel, and visited the schools in Leipzig, Prague, and Vienna. In 1817, he took over a new school in Königsberg. (134, p. 36) In 1827, he published a booklet, setting out his ideas and the results of his studies and observations of the various schools for deaf children in Europe. He studied the French system carefully, and felt that the greatest mistake made by de l'Épée, and compounded by Sicard, was in attributing to signs a perfection and refinement of expression which they did not possess. He considered the use of signs vague and confusing, and thought they only presented an added obstacle to the deaf pupil in his learning of his native language. (42, Vol. II, pp. 4-8)

HOLLAND

Henry Daniel Guyot was born November 25, 1753, in Frois-Fontaines, a village in the southern part of what became the province of Limburg, in the Netherlands. His family was of French origin, but fled from France in 1700 to escape persecution for their religious faith. Henry's father was a medical doctor. He died when the boy was three, so that he was forced to become independent while still very young. He was a brilliant student and of a pleasant and tolerant disposition.

On a visit to Paris in 18784, he met de l'Épée, and became interested in teaching deaf children. His first pupils were a Jewish boy and a Christian girl. His success with these two led to his founding of The Groningen Institution for Deaf-Mutes in 1790.

Guyot's first methods were largely the manual methods of the French system, but he also taught speech as an extra to some of his pupils. Later he was influenced by his sons to attempt more speech, so that through most of his lifetime, he used the "old Dutch" or mixed method.

He died at the age of 74, January 10, 1828, with his reputation for good and his institution for deaf both firmly established. (26)[a]

In 1790, the year the Institution at Groningen was founded, triplets were born to the Guyot family. Charles, the eldest of these sons, became his father's successor in the school. (26)

ENGLAND

The most outstanding name in England, concerned with the education of the deaf, was that of a Scotsman, Thomas Braidwood. He was born in 1715 and educated at Edinburgh University. (8,b, p.66)

After teaching in a grammar school at Hamilton, he opened a school of mathematics in Edinburgh. In 1760, Alexander Shirreff, a wealthy merchant of Craigleith, brought him his son Charles, deafened at the age of three, and begged Braidwood to teach him to write. Braidwood was intrigued by the challenge and, knowing nothing of previous manual methods, began the boy's instruction in the way that seemed to him to be natural. He taught him to talk. The speech vocabulary thus acquired by the boy was fixed in his memory by means of lipreading and writing. (14; 175,a)

His success with Shirreff encouraged Braidwood to accept another boy, born deaf, the son of Dr. John Douglas, a physician of London. In January, 1766, he placed an advertisement in the Scots Magazine, in which a friend, identified only as "J. H.," described his work with the two deaf boys and their accomplishments.

---

[a] All the Dutch material in this book was translated and interpreted by Annetta Aarsen de Graff of Lisse, Holland.

The first (who lost his hearing about three years of age), son to Alexander Shirreff, Esq. . . . , a lad of fifteen, who has been for some time under Mr. Braidwood's care, reads any English book distinctly, and understands both the meaning and the grammatical construction of the passages which he reads. He answers questions put to him with great readiness, and his manner of pronouncing is articulate and distinct. He understands what is spoken by persons with whom he is familiar, and even by anyone who speaks distinct and slow, from the motion of their lips. . . . He writes with elegance; is throughly master of arithmetic, book-keeping, and geography; and is no inconsiderable proficient in drawing. He is to be bred a merchant, and it is thought he will excell in that business.

His other pupil, who was born deaf, son to Dr. John Douglas, physician of London, is a boy of thirteen. He had been only four months under Dr. Braidwood's care, but his progress is remarkable; and in some things, particularly the tone of his voice, and his manner of articulation, he excels the former; owing chiefly to the superior skill which Mr. Braidwood has acquired by experience. (175,a)

On July 28, 1767, a similar letter described more successful pupils:

Mr. Braidwood has several deaf pupils at present, who are all making surprising progress in their education. . . . A boy of nine who has been eight months with him reads any English book slowly and pronounces distinctly, so that anyone who hears him understands with ease what he says. . . . Two young ladies, one of nine and the other of seven, . . . can pronounce all the letters and simple syllables correctly and distinctly.

Mr. Braidwood . . . thinks he may undertake to teach anyone of a tolerable genius in the space of about three years to speak and to read distinctly, to write readily, to perform the common rules of arithmetic. . . . and to have a tolerable notion of the principles of religion. He has had deaf pupils from twenty-five to seven years of age; he finds the younger they are, they pronounce the easier. He has likewise had considerable success in correcting the defects of persons who stutter, or have other impediments in their speech. (175,b)

Two years later, Braidwood made an effort to secure public support for the education of the deaf. Another letter was published in the Scots Magazine, July 15, 1769:

Mr. Braidwood, writing master in Edinburgh, claims the notice of the public . . . as having discovered a method by which he is able to teach the deaf and dumb to speak, read, and write, and cipher, etc. However astonishing this feat may appear, it is sufficiently known to many who have attended at the public examinations of his pupils, both here and at London. . . .

Mr. Braidwood has at present several deaf pupils . . . but it is to be regretted that he has been obliged to refuse above thirty deaf persons . . . as he can only teach a few at the same time, which of necessity renders the expense of this kind of education greater than some parents can afford.

In order to render Mr. Braidwood's art universally useful, two things are necessary. The first is, that he shall communicate his skill to three or four ingenious young men, who may assist and succeed him in this business; and the second is that some kind of fund be established under the direction of proper managers, to be applied for defraying the expenses of educating such whose parents are unable to take that burden upon them.

N.B. Most of those who have applied could afford part of the expense.

By this means so useful an art would be preserved, and no unfortunate subject be deprived of the benefit arising from it.

Mr. Braidwood has generously declared his readiness to communicate his skill to others upon the above plan; and in an age distinguished by so many public charities, and so ready to encourage every invention in arts or science, a fund sufficient for the purpose might be obtained, by an application to his Majesty, or otherwise. . . .

The design of this letter is, to excite the generous and compassionate among the nobility and gentry, to inquire into the facts already mentioned, and to afford themselves the opportunity of patronizing the scheme, so truly charitable and so useful to society. If Mr. Braidwood receives no public encouragement, he will be obliged to move in the same confined task as hitherto, and teach only deaf persons who can afford the expense; and when he dies his valuable gift will probably die with him. (175,c)

Apparently Braidwood received no public encouragement. After this rebuff, he withdrew within the limits of his own family, making his techniques a family secret, and placing under bond of secrecy anyone to whom he taught his methods.

His school and his reputation grew rapidly, in spite of the lack of public support. He soon took in with him his nephew, John Braidwood, to assist in the growing task.

Noted travelers visited the school, and wrote of it in glowing terms as one of the wonders of Scotland. Thomas Pennant, the author and traveler, visited him in 1772. In his book *Tour of Scotland,* he described the skill of Braidwood's pupils in "seeing our words and speaking by imitation." In 1774, Lord Monboddo included in his work *Of the Origin and Progess of Language* an account of Charles Shirreff, who had been Braidwood's first pupil. (80, p. 23)

Samuel Johnson, while exploring the Western Islands of Scotland in 1772, included the school in his itinerary and was much impressed by what he saw. He wrote a detailed description of it in his account of the journey:

There is one subject of philosophical curiosity to be found in Edinburgh, which no other city has to shew; a college of deaf and dumb, who are taught to speak, to read, to write, and to practice arithmetic, by a gentleman whose name is Braidwood. (80, p. 380)

Johnson referred to previous teachers of the deaf, some of whom he had seen, but added that,

the improvement of Mr. Braidwood's pupils is wonderful. They not only speak, write, and understand what is written, but if he that speaks looks towards them and modifies his organs by distinct and full utterance, they know so well what is spoken that it is an expression scarcely figurative to say they hear with the eye. (80, p. 381)

He concluded with the warm comment that

It was pleasing to see one of the most desperate of human calamities capable of so much help. (80, p. 383)

In 1780, Braidwood received a pupil from America. Francis Green, a citizen of Boston, brought his eight-year-old son Charles to him. Induced by "the tender concern of an only parent for an only son," the father lived in England for a number of years in order to be near his motherless boy. Before he returned to the United States, Green published an account of his son's education, which is one of our best expositions of the Braidwood method. (64)

By 1783, Braidwood felt that his school had prospered sufficiently to justify moving it to a more populous center. So he took the school and his assistant to Hackney, near London. Their first address there was Grove House, Mare Street. It was here that John Braidwood married a daughter of his uncle Thomas Braidwood. (75, p. 148) The identical names and the relationship of John Braidwood's sons to his father-in-law caused considerable confusion among later historians. They had a tendency to assume that, since the boys were the grandsons of Thomas Braidwood, John Braidwood was his son. He has been identified, however, as his nephew. (8,b, p. 70; 140, p. 65)

The school prospered in its new location, so much so that a year later it was necessary to bring in another nephew, Joseph Watson, to help with the work. John Braidwood died in 1798, leaving the control of the school to his widow and Watson, until his two young sons, Thomas and John, should be of age.

The first detailed account we have of the Braidwood methods of teaching was in the book by Francis Green, published in London in 1783. He took for his title the Braidwood motto, *Vox Oculis Subjec-*

ta (The Voice made subject to the Eyes). Or, as he himself interpreted it, "as it may be Englished, the voice made visible." (64, p. 23) He added the descriptive title:

> Dissertation on the most curious and important Art of Imparting Speech and the Knowledge of Language to the Naturally Deaf and (consequently) Dumb; with a particular account of the Academy of Messrs. Braidwood of Edinburgh and a proposal to perpetuate the benefits thereof.

The book was signed, quite simply, "By a Parent."

In the Introduction, Green gave this discussion of the current philosophy of deafness:

> The principal channel through which instruction and knowledge (the source of infinite pleasure) are usually conveyed to the mind is the ear. This, by some internal, unaccountable misformation or derangement (of their organs of hearing) is blocked up forever! To them all nature wears a solemn silence; the consequence is that speech, that mark of humanity, that peculiar ornament and dignity, which chiefly distinguishes man from the brute creation, is unattainable in the common way, it being, evidently, by the imitation of the sounds which we hear that mankind ordinarily acquire the art or the faculty of speech. (64, pp. 8-9)

He paid the same tribute to the atmosphere of the school as Samuel Johnson had done previously.

> A mistake or prejudice respecting the methods of teaching articulation I find hath been imbibed by some upon a supposition that harsh and severe methods were privately used in order to enforce exertions contrary to their natural disposition and inclinations, and such a rigid discipline as is sometimes practiced upon persons deprived of reason. . . .
>
> Nothing can possibly be more remote from a true description of their methods, for the most kind and affectionate mode is practiced, much more tender, ingratiating, and consistent with the true art of governing the human mind, and making learning a pleasure than I ever saw at any other school. The behavior of the pupils is the most convincing proof imaginable of this; they enter punctually the school room, with an eagerness that shows they really love their learning, not regarding it (as young persons in general do) as a hardship or imposition, but as an indulgence. (64, pp. 145-146)

In the school, all were lodged under the same roof with the teachers. The boys and girls had separate living quarters, but were brought together in the classrooms. Their ages ranged from five to twenty. Those, however, who are taken in hand when young, before the organs grow stiff and rigid from want of use, generally speak most plainly and pleasantly.

Five years was considered necessary

for understanding of their own language, so as to read, write, and speak it with ease.

Green also quoted,

Mr. Braidwood, who hath often acknowledged to me that his success, in consequence of new discoveries, made in the course of teaching hath greatly exceeded what was at first his highest or most sanguine expectations. (64, pp. 140-141)

He further described the methods used, saying that the tutors kept in no fixed seat, but were constantly moving about among the pupils, giving help wherever it was needed. The only instrument used was

a small, round piece of silver, the size of a tobacco pipe, flatted at one end, with a ball (as large as a marble) at the other; by means of which the tongue is gently placed, at first, in various positions respectively proper for forming the articulations of the different letters and syllables, until they acquire (as we all do in learning speech) by habit, the proper method. (64, p. 147)

He told the story of his own son. The boy was either born deaf or deafened in early infancy. His hearing loss was discovered by accident at the age of six months. At the age of eight years, when he was first brought to school, he

could not produce nor distinguish articulate vocal sounds, nor had any idea of the meaning of words, either spoken, in writing, or in print.

In May, 1781, his father paid him his first visit at the school. The boy greeted him in speech and asked questions about his family. His father gave him a letter from his sister "couched in simplest terms," which Charles read aloud, interpreting his understanding to his father by gestures. He recited the Lord's Prayer. He also recited some prayer forms unfamiliar to his father, which he wrote down at his son's dictation, as proof of the intelligibility of his speech. (64, p. 149)

Part III of the book was entitled, "A proposal to Perpetuate and Extend the Benefits of this Important Art."

Green repeated the arguments that Braidwood had used in

Scotland in 1769:

> To render this art universally useful, it is necessary that some ingenious young men should be instructed and qualified to assist and succeed the present professors, and that a fund should be established under the direction of proper managers, to be applied to the purpose of the education of those whose parents are altogether unable to defray such expense, and to assist others who can afford a part but not the whole, by which means all the deaf, however scattered, might be collected and taught.
>
> Messrs. Braidwood have repeatedly declared their readiness to undertake to qualify a sufficient number of young men for the execution of such a plan. (64, pp. 180-181)

He had no doubt that the funds could easily be raised by charity, by private donation, and by government subsidy. But Green, also, received no immediate response in England.

Upon his return to the United States, Green made every effort to encourage the establishment of education for the deaf in his own country. Even though Charles died in 1787, at the age of fifteen, his father continued his interest in the work. (43,b, p. 92) In 1803, he solicited the help of the ministers in the community, and conducted a census of the deaf in New England. Only seventy-five could be definitely listed, and it was estimated that there were five hundred in the United States. Green strongly urged the need for a school, writing articles for the public magazines to plead the cause of deaf children in the United States. But, for the time being, his efforts fell on sterile ground. (20, p. 386)

Joseph Watson, born 1765, was the second nephew of Thomas Braidwood to join him in the family profession. Educated by his uncle at Hackney, he decided, in 1784, to continue in the work of teaching the deaf.

In 1792, the need for support for the education of the deaf was again brought to the attention of the public. The Reverend John Townshend, a Congregational minister at Bermondsey, became interested in the project through a Mrs. Creasy, whose son was a pupil of the Braidwoods. He organized a committee charged with the education of indigent deaf. In November of the same year this committee opened a school for deaf in Grange Road, Bermondsey, where they installed six children, three boys and three girls, with Joseph Watson as their teacher. Watson did not receive a salary, but was expected to make a profit on his contracts for school supplies and on any fee-paying pupils he took in. The committee provided maintenance for the charity children. The one private pupil, who enrolled at the opening of the school, paid tuition and lived with

Watson instead of with the other children. Thus the schools for the deaf in England were established on a charity and asylum basis. (8,b, p. 68; 75, pp. 148-149)

At the death of Thomas Braidwood in 1806, Watson apparently considered himself released from the family bond of secrecy. In 1809, he published a two-volume work called *Instruction of the Deaf and Dumb, A Theoretical and Practical View of the Means by which They are Taught to Speak and Understand.*

He stated that his principles were the same as those founded by his uncle. He did not believe in the methodical signs of de l'Épée, considering them fanciful and useless. He recommended beginning with articulation, first combining speech elements into syllables, then into words. From there he went on to writing and reading. As a means of communication until oral language could be established, he accepted natural gestures and signs, and recommended a two-handed alphabet which is still in use in England today. Numerous copperplate illustrations throughout the book showed the most common objects necessary for the beginner's vocabulary. (136,a; 184)

By 1810, Watson's school had seventy pupils. Spacious new quarters were opened for them on Kent Road, and the teaching of a number of trades was introduced. Although patrons of the school were encouraged to buy from the school shops, much of this department had later to be abandoned because it was too expensive.

By 1820, the number of pupils in the school had risen to two hundred. In spite of the rising costs, the children were well looked after. The committee in charge of their maintenance found the money somewhere, by means of charitable donations, to keep up with the children's needs.

Joseph Watson died in 1829, a comparatively rich man. The committee had never paid him more than a nominal salary. He made his money from the tuition of the private pupils and the contracts for school supplies. The committee was well enough pleased with their bargain to appoint Watson's son, Thomas, as his father's successor. (75, p. 177)

After the elder Thomas Braidwood moved his first school from Edinburgh to Hackney, Scotland was left without a permanent school for the deaf until 1810. Then the Edinburgh Institute was opened in Henderson Row. Administered by the same committee that looked after the schools in England, the headship of the school in Edinburgh was given to John Braidwood, son of John and grandson of Thomas Braidwood.

The magic of the family name was not enough to insure his capability. John was an alcoholic and irresponsible. In two years, he left for America. There is a strong suggestion in the accounts of the young man's life that the emigration was necessitated by his own behavior. (8,b, p. 70; 75, p. 178; 140)

After his departure, Robert Kinniburgh was appointed in his place.

At Birmingham General Hospital, in Birmingham, England, there was a young doctor, de Lys, who was of a refugee family from Brittany. In the course of his practice, he became interested in a deaf girl who came under his care. Hoping to help her to an education, he made contact with the Braidwoods. His interest in the problem grew to such an extent that he demonstrated to the Birmingham Philosophical Society the little speech he, himself, had managed to teach the girl. Under his inspiration, funds were raised to start the Birmingham Institution for the Instruction of Deaf and Dumb Children.

At the beginning, this was a day school for fifteen children. Thomas Braidwood, son of John and grandson of the elder Thomas Braidwood, was appointed head of the school. It was moved to larger quarters "in the country" near Edgebarton, in 1813, as an asylum for 175 children. Thomas Braidwood held the position of director, with integrity and efficiency, until his death in 1825.

After the death of Thomas Braidwood, the committee appointed a Swiss named Louis du Puget to the position. He was well versed in the French system of teaching the deaf, and introduced finger spelling and methodical signs. With him, the Braidwood dynasty in England's schools for the deaf was ended. (75, p. 163)

UNITED STATES

In the United States, early references were made in historical papers to isolated cases of deaf persons who were given some attention. In 1679 there was a deaf and dumb boy in Rowley, Massachusetts, whose name was Isaac Kilbourne. A man named Philip Nelson was reported to have cured him. Those were the days of belief in witchcraft, and the ministers of the community were called in to investigate the possibility that witches had been invoked. It is not clear whether this was a successful effort at teaching a deaf boy, or whether an actual cure was claimed. (11, p. 385)

A hundred years later, another deaf boy was reported in Virginia. From 1773 to 1776, John Edge was in the classes of John Harrower, a schoolmaster at Fredericksburg. Harrower referred to the boy in his diary. (20, p. 383)

As the country grew in national consciousness, more and more account was taken in the writings of the day concerning the deaf and their need for education. In 1790, the Massachusetts Magazine published an account of a visit to the school for the deaf in Paris, and expressed the hope that similar schools might be created in the United States. Green's Vox Oculis Subjecta was reviewed in the Boston Magazine in 1784 and 1785. In 1793, Dr. William Thornton published Cadmus: A Treatise on the Elements of Written Language, with an appendix called Essay on a Mode of Teaching the Deaf, or Surd, and Consequently Dumb, to Speak. (184)

In 1810, the Reverend John Stanford, who was chaplain of the Humane and Criminal Institutions of New York, discovered several deaf children living in the New York almshouse, completely untaught. He tried to teach them what he could, buying slates and pencils for them to use, and began to work towards a school for deaf children. His efforts finally resulted in the establishment of the New York Institution for the Deaf and Dumb, which was opened in 1818, with sixty children. The city gave ten thousand dollars and guaranteed a part of the tax on lotteries as income for the school. About half the children were admitted as charity cases, while the remainder paid some tuition. This school later became known as the New York School for the Deaf. (20, p. 388)

At first, deaf children from well-to-do families in America were sent to Europe for their education. The nephew of President Monroe went to school in Paris. (20, p. 388) The story has already been told of Charles Green of Boston, who was educated in the Braidwood school.

In Chesterfield County, Virginia, a Major Thomas Bolling had three deaf children, John, Thomas, and Mary, who were sent to England to be educated by the Braidwoods. A letter written by his hearing son, William, dated December 10, 1841, and addressed to the Reverend Joseph D. Tyler, then principal of the Virginia Institution, gave this account of them:

> It may be interesting to you to be informed of the education of my two brothers, John and Thomas, and that of my sister Mary, who were all born in that situation. John Bolling, the oldest, was sent by my father in the year 1771 to Edinburgh, and placed under the care and tuition of Thomas Braidwood. Thomas and Mary Bolling followed him in 1775. They all remained at his school during the Revolutionary War, and all returned to "Cobbs" in Chesterfield County, Virginia, the residence of my father, Major Thomas Bolling, in July, 1783.
> John died about three months after his return.

Thomas's acquirements were most extraordinary. He was a ready penman, of nice, discriminating judgement, of scrupulous integrity; in all of his transactions his intelligence and tact in communication were such as to attract the attention, entertain, and amuse every company in which he associated, with the manners of a most polished gentleman; his articulation so perfect that his family and friends and the servants understood him in conversation or in reading aloud.

My sister's acquirements were equal to his, though her voice was not so pleasant, yet she was cheerful, intelligent, entertaining, and industrious. She died in 1826; my brother, Thomas, in 1836, in the 70th year of his age. (144, p. 3)

William Bolling passed on the family deafness to his children, William Albert and Mary. As he was considering the necessity of sending William Albert to England for his education, young John Braidwood arrived in Washington. The Representative from Virginia, who was in Washington at the time, and a friend of the Bolling family, immediately informed them of the young man's arrival.

Bolling invited Braidwood to visit him, and he came to Virginia in May, 1812. He informed his host that his plans were to rent a suitable house in Baltimore and open a school there. He was, he said, cut off from receiving remittances from London because the United States had declared war on Great Britain. But several gentlemen in Philadelphia and Baltimore had engaged his services for several scholars and advanced him $600 each to establish the school. So Bolling also gave him $600, with the understanding that the school was to open by July 1. He also went to Richmond with him, where an advertisement for the school was placed in the Richmond Enquirer.

The next time Bolling heard from Braidwood he was in New York, in prison for debt. Bolling sent another $600 for his release and brought the young man into his own home.

In November of the same year, Braidwood began the education of the Bolling children. Bolling at first described him as

faithful and diligent, exhibiting unequalled evidence of his qualifications in his profession.

He was much gratified by his son's progress until the summer of 1813, when his military duties took him to Norfolk for six months.

From this time on he (Braidwood) began to relax and on my return had almost abandoned his duties. (144, p. 2)

However, the school was successful enough that other parents were seeking admission for their children. So, in 1815, the school was moved to "Cobbs," where Bolling turned over to Braidwood the family estate, with a large house and furniture, in addition to a salary for his teaching.

But, in 1817, Braidwood suddenly left Virginia and went to New York, where he "did nothing," according to Bolling. A year later he was back in Virginia, "penniless, friendless, and scarcely decently clad," and went once more to Bolling for assistance. This time a new school was opened in Manchester, Virginia, with the Reverend John Kirkpatrick[a] in charge (20, p. 389), and Braidwood as his assistant. For six months his conduct was entirely satisfactory. Then his old habits overcame him again.

Young William Albert Bolling seemed to progress well in the new school. He kept an exercise book of daily compositions. One of his little stories was quoted thus:

> This morning John Hancock caught Mrs. McRae's little black boy Peter and brought him into the porch. Mr. Harris took him and put him in the closet and shut the door. Mr. Harris then went and got a rod and went into the closet and whipped Peter for throwing stones. Peter promised he would not throw any more stones, and Mr. Harris told him to put on his clothes and go home and be a good boy. (43,b, p. 96)

The little story gives evidence of the excellent language teaching in the Braidwood method. The sentence structures are accurate and normal, and the incidents clearly expressed.

On June 25, 1818, this comment appeared in the boy's notebook:

> It is five minutes past three o'clock. Mr. Braidwood has not come into school.

This was apparently Braidwood's last connection with the school. It was carried on for a year or two longer by Kirkpatrick before the work was abandoned. Braidwood died in 1819, "a victim of intemperance,"[b] (140, p. 65; 144, p. 3)

Credit for the permanent establishment of education for the deaf in the United States has been given to Thomas Hopkins Gallaudet.

Born in Philadelphia, December 10, 1787, of a French Huguenot family, he moved with his family to Hartford, Connecticut, as a young man, in 1800. He attended the Hartford grammar school and graduated from Yale College in 1805. A brilliant and talented student, he began the study of law, but the condition of his health

[a] Best makes the name Kilpatrick.
[b] Other authorities place his death in 1820.

would not allow him to continue. In 1808, he was a tutor at Yale College, a position which he held for two years. Then he took a business commission in order to be able to travel for his health. In 1812, he took up the study of theology at Andover, Massachusetts, and was licensed to preach in 1814, at the age of twenty-seven.

It was during the winter of 1814-1815 that he met his first deaf pupil. Home from college because of his health, he noticed the little deaf daughter of his neighbor, Dr. Cogswell, playing in her father's garden with other children. He was much interested in the little girl, then nine years old, and tried his hand at teaching her. By writing a word, and showing her the object, he found that she learned to read quite readily. The first word he taught her in this fashion was "hat."

This little girl, Alice Cogswell, was born in 1805, the daughter of Dr. Mason Fitch Cogswell. At the age of two years and three months, she was ill with "spotted fever" (a common name for cerebro-spinal meningitis). This illness took her hearing, after which she gradually lost her speech as well.

Her father was reluctant to send his little daughter to Europe for her education, and hoped instead to set up some means of teaching deaf children in the United States. He gathered together a group of clergymen, as had Francis Green before, and with their help took a census of the deaf of educable age in Connecticut. Eighty such persons were found, and it was estimated from this survey that there should be 400 in New England and "upwards of 2000" in the United States.

Meanwhile, Gallaudet had continued his interest in Alice Cogswell. He studied a publication of Sicard's, which Dr. Cogswell had in his library, and began to combine signs and the manual alphabet with writing in his teaching. He also persuaded the Cogswells to secure the services of Lydia Huntley as Alice's governess.

On April 13, 1815, Dr. Cogswell called together ten of his friends and neighbors—merchants, educators, business men of the community—in his home. He presented to them the need for education for deaf children in the United States, as proved by his survey, and proposed the opening of such a school at Hartford.

Enough money was subscribed immediately to send a teacher to study in Europe. The group deliberated on methods, and decided that their representative should go to England and study the oral method of the Braidwoods.

It was not surprising that their choice of a teacher fell on the young man who had taken such a constructive interest in little Alice. Gallaudet was offered the position. He hesitated at first, having by this time planned his own career, but he soon allowed himself to be persuaded.

On May 25, 1815, Thomas Hopkins Gallaudet sailed for England, and landed at Liverpool, June 25.

Once in England, he met unexpected difficulties. He applied to Thomas Braidwood at Birmingham and also Joseph Watson at Old Kent Road for admission to their schools. He proposed to remain a few months to learn their method, then combine it with Sicard's manual method, choosing what he judged best from both. When this was not acceptable to the Braidwoods, he requested that they release Kinniburgh, in the Edinburgh school, from his obligation of secrecy to the family, that he might learn from him.

Thomas Braidwood conferred with his mother at Hackney. It could hardly have been a pleasing idea to the Braidwood family. They were at bitter odds with the French manual method. Besides, brother John was at that moment in the United States, attempting to establish an oral school for deaf. So Gallaudet's proposition was denied.

Watson then made an offer to send one of his assistants to America to assist in establishing the proposed school. This did not suit Gallaudet's plans. He felt that such a teacher would be "wedded to Dr. Watson's mode," while he wished to be free to work out his own methods as he judged best, combining what he thought to be

> the peculiar advantages of both the French and English modes of instruction. For there are considerable differences between them. (57, p. 66)

The sub-committee of the London school then proposed to Gallaudet that he establish himself in that school for three years. They offered to employ him as an assistant at the regular salary for that length of time. His duties were to keep him

> with the pupils from seven o'clock in the morning till eight in the evening, and also with the pupils in their hours of recreation. (57, p. 66)

This proposition was definitely not to Gallaudet's liking. His letters home to his sponsors were full of protests, not only about the Braidwoods, but also about the sponsors, who had not, he felt, allowed him enough money to travel with dignity.

He employed some of his time, while he was waiting for the results of his negotiations with the Braidwoods, in preaching from Scottish pulpits.

Meanwhile his little friend Alice Cogswell, who was continuing her studies at home with Lydia Huntley, cheered him with her quaint letters:

Hartford, Wednesday, October 11, 1815.

My dear Sir:—

I remember story Miss Huntley tell me. Old many years Mr. Colt little boy Name man Peter Colt very much curls. Little boy hair Oh! very beautiful mama lap little boy comb curl love to see O beautiful. Morning long man preacher coat make wigs very beautiful man say come back little boy scissors cut hair while hair curls all in heap make wig am very much glad proud little-little boy head very cold mama tie handkerchief warm, tears no more mama very sorry. I hope my hair never cut make wigs—This morning study all in school away Geography all beautiful all very beautiful very still very good noise no—the Play no. Miss Huntley work and two go Norwich all school come not—me very sorry come back little while—O all very glad O beautiful—I love you very much—

Your affectionate
Alice Cogswell

Alice's father wrote to Gallaudet at the same time, describing the circumstances of his daughter's letter. Her teacher had told her the story in sign language, and Alice related it in writing, naturally using the same word order given by the signs. (57, pp. 86-87)

The lack of sentence structure and verb tenses is a direct translation from the sign language.

It happened that at this same time the Abbé Sicard was on a lecture tour in London, accompanied by two of his most famous pupils, Massieu and Clerc. Gallaudet went to see the demonstration of the accomplishments of these pupils. He also described to Sicard his mission and the difficulty he was having in accomplishing it. Sicard promptly invited him to Paris for a visit at his school.

Gallaudet broke off negotiations with the Braidwoods and crossed over to Paris on March 9, 1816. He was at once placed in training, attending classes, and receiving private lessons from Massieu.

In June, Gallaudet decided to return to America. Laurent Clerc, a deaf pupil who had risen to be an assistant teacher, offered to accompany him and help in establishing the new school at Hartford. (8,b, pp. 94-95; 14; 57, p. 102; 43,b, p. 98-103)

The first problem facing Gallaudet on his return to the United States was money to establish the school. Accompanied by Laurent Clerc, Gallaudet visited various cities to plead the cause of education for the deaf. Clerc communicated with hearing people by means of writing, on a slate which he carried with him. He had good command of English and French, and made a good impression. In October 1816, the legislature of Connecticut appropriated $5,000 for the enterprise,

> which is believed to have been the first appropriation of public money made in America in behalf of a benevolent institution. (57, p. 116)

Private donations continued to add to the fund until $17,000 had been accumulated.

On April 15, 1817, the school was opened with seven pupils. In July, 1817, the first annual report of the American Asylum for the Deaf was published at Hartford by the order of the directors.

The report opened with a list of the names of the pupils in the order of their admission to the school. There were twenty-one names, and that of Alice Cogswell was first on the list. The report continued with a glowing picture of the happiness and progress of the pupils, along with a history of the founding of the school. (190,a)

The second report, a year later, added forty new names to the list of pupils, and included some letters written by a few of the more advanced students. (190,b)

The third report made the comment that the teachers' residence was under the same roof with the pupils, so that they might have constant communication. Four steps in teaching were described. Signs were taught to the teachers by Clerc, but were kept simple, natural pantomime, rather than the methodical signs of de l'Épée. This was the first means of communication with the children. Second, more conventional signs were introduced and taught. Third, the manual alphabet was taught, and used to spell words. Fourth, writing was taught, in connection with the manual alphabet, and used for language expression.

By this time articulation had been completely abandoned. The methods of Braidwood were referred to as "parlor tricks" with no meaning, and "entitled to rank little higher than training starlings or parrots." (190,c, pp. 6-8)

On the campus of the present American School for the Deaf at Hartford stands a beautiful statue of Gallaudet and Alice Cogswell. He is seated, with his head bent to her small one. Alice stands in the crook of his arm, her head thrown back to lift her face to him. Each of them is holding up a hand, clenched in the form of the letter A of the manual alphabet.

At first the school at Hartford had to depend heavily on private contributions for continuing support. For this pupose, pupils were taken on demonstration tours to church assemblies and before the legislatures of neighboring states.

It was soon evident that this educational movement was of national significance. In 1819, Laurent Clerc was sent to Washington to solicit help from Congress. Henry Clay, who was then Speaker of the House, took a favorable interest in the project. An act was passed, appropriating 23,000 acres of public land for the school. Eventually about $300,000 was realized from this grant.

Other states began immediately to take account of the deaf children within their own borders. Some sent their children to the Hartford school at public expense, until such time as they found it practical to open their own schools. Others immediately set about establishing state schools for deaf children, each within the borders of its own commonwealth.

Thus, education for the deaf was established in the United States, from the beginning, as a public responsibility.

Sophia Fowler, deaf from birth, was admitted to the Hartford school in the spring of 1817. Her name was fifteenth on the list of pupils enrolled. On August 29, 1821, she was married to Thomas Hopkins Gallaudet. (57, pp. 144-146)

Gallaudet remained as principal of the American Asylum for thirteen years. In April, 1830, he forwarded a petition to the directors of the school, in which he requested to be released from his teaching duties so that he might have full time to give to administration and to further the progress of the school. He had always spent six hours a day in classroom teaching, in addition to his duties as principal.

The directors agreed to grant the request. But the assistant instructors were bitterly resentful of the added power this would seem to give Gallaudet over them. When they realized that their attitude was driving Gallaudet to complete resignation, they withdrew their objections. By this time it was too late. Galluadet's health would no longer allow him to continue under the constant strain. He resigned, and left the school in October, 1830.

He continued his interest in other philanthropic institutions and welfare organizations. He wrote religious books for children. He accepted a position as chaplain of the Connecticut Retreat for the Insane.

Late in 1849, the house in which the Gallaudet family lived on Leffingwell Street, in Hartford, was to be sold. Gallaudet wished to own his home, and he wanted a house on Buckingham Street, closer to the Retreat. His daily walks to and from the Institution were too long. The cost of this house was $2,500.

Seth Terry, at that time Commissioner of Funds to the American Asylum, was an old friend of Gallaudet. He well knew how poorly the principal had been paid for his services, during his years at the school. So Terry proposed to the Board of Directors, in February, 1850, that the school give Gallaudet $2,000 toward the purchase of his house. This was presented to him, along with a purse of $500, made up by his friends.

On April first, he received the deed to the house, and on April ninth, the Gallaudet family moved into their new quarters.

On September 27 of the same year, a testimonal assembly was held in the Center church of Hartford, by Gallaudet's old pupils. Tributes were paid to both Gallaudet and Clerc for their years of service for the education of the deaf. Each of them was presented with a silver pitcher and tray.

Gallaudet died at Hartford, September 10, 1851, highly honored, both in his own country and abroad. (57; 153a)

The eighteenth century saw the establishment of permanent schools for the education of the deaf in all the major countries of the western world. From the outset, the major purpose of these schools was educational. The thought of providing an asylum from the outside world was also implicit in all but the German approach to the project, but nowhere was the basic purpose of instruction submerged by the welfare aspect of the problem.

There was no longer any turning back, in the education of the deaf, as had happened in previous centuries. From now on, their place as an educational responsibility was firmly established.

Chapter 8

The Trend of Progress

(1825-1880)

As education entered the nineteenth century, the thoughts of leading educators settled more and more on the child, instead of exclusively on the subject matter to be taught. Education, instead of being purely a preparation for the future became, at least in part, a way of living for the present. The concept of a program of learning geared to the natural developmental progress of the child began to take root.

Among the leaders of education for deaf children, in this era, one of the first who attempted to draw their pattern of educational and social training closer to the normal, was Johann Baptist Graser (1766-1841), a native of Bavaria. He received little attention, at first. But after the retreat of Napoleon's armies, there was an upsurge of national feeling and a tendency to discard anything that was French and return to German ways. Graser had never accepted the use of signs in teaching deaf children, but maintained the old German techniques of oral teaching. By the time the new national emphasis brought his work forward, Graser was fifty-five, and had a background of experience that gave his words authority.

He maintained that a great fault of the education of the deaf was its isolation. At his instigation, departments were set up in normal schools and seminaries to train all teachers in methods of teaching deaf children. Those who did not care to undertake a complete study of the field, were sent for a special six weeks course of concentrated instruction at one of these special training centers.

In 1821, Graser opened an experimental school for the deaf as a department of an ordinary school in Bayreuth. His plan was to give the children a year and a half to two years of special training, then incorporate them into the regular classes, whose teachers were expected to be trained to teach the deaf children along with the hearing. (8,b, p. 60; 152, p. 106; 75, pp. 177-178)

In 1829, he published *The Deaf-Mute restored to Humanity by Visible and Spoken Speech,* in which he described his philosophy for giving a normal educational life to deaf children. He was quoted by a later historian, thus:

> The only way of restoring the deaf-mute to society, from which he is excluded by reason of his infirmity, is to give him the power of conversing like hearing persons. So far a great obstacle in the way of obtaining this desired end is that the deaf-mutes were required to learn two languages at the same time, namely the finger spelling and the spoken language. The greater value has always been attached to the former, the consequence the latter has never been perfectly mastered. The pupils have learned to speak a few words and phrases, but they have never been able to use speech as a means of social intercourse. (68, p. 125)

As first, the idea was accepted with enthusiasm, and classes for deaf children were made a part of the public school system in many German states. But not enough allowance had been made for the slower pace at which the deaf children were acquiring their education, and, after a few years, the system was gradually abandoned.

Victor August Jäger was the founder and head of the Institution for the Deaf-Mute and Blind, at Gmünd, in Würtemburg, Germany. In 1825 he published a book called *Guide to the Instruction of Deaf-Mute Children.* This book was a return to the use of speech for deaf children, and a vigorous attack on the use of methodical signs and the manual alphabet. Its publication did much to discourage the combined method and restore oralism in the German schools. It was used as a guide for German teachers of deaf children until it was replaced by the textbooks of Hill, about twenty years later. (8,b, p. 57)

Every effort was made to retain a normal environment for the deaf child. Jäger told the story of a little girl who lost her hearing at four years of age. She still spoke the dialect of her district at twenty, although she had received no other schooling than that of her local village school, which she entered at the age of seven. How severe was the hearing loss, was not reported. But the story illustrated the point that a child who lost his hearing did not also need to lose his speech, nor his normal contact with his environment. The book was called, *Concerning the Manner by which Blind and Deaf-Mute Children Shall be Restored to their Place.* (79)

One of the greatest of the German teachers of the deaf was Friedrich Moritz Hill. Born December 8, 1805, at Reichenbach, near Breslau, Germany, he was the son of a musician. He showed considerable musical talent, and enjoyed playing with his father's groups of musicians. His father was delighted and wanted him to continue a musical career. But his mother protested that he was too young to play all night for dances, and wanted him to be a teacher.

He followed his mother's inclinations, although finding a good deal of time on the side to play for churches and schools. Some of his training as a teacher was received under Johann Heinrich Pestalozzi.

In May of 1828, while studying in Berlin, he heard an announcement concerning a course for teaching deaf mutes. This caught his interest in such earnest that in 1830 he entered the old Heinicke institute at Weissenfels, where he remained until his death in 1874. (108)

He spent his life teaching and writing in the interests of the education of the deaf. His books were published in rapid order. Following is a partial list:

> 1838, *Guide to Deaf-Mute Instruction*
> 1839, *Complete Guide to the Instruction of Deaf-Mute Children, in Mechanical Speech, Lipreading, Reading, and Writing, for Public School Teachers*
> 1840, *Guide to the Instruction of the Deaf and Dumb for Pastors and Teachers*
> 1866, *Present Condition of the System of Deaf-Mute Instruction in Germany* (73)

Hill applied the principles of Pestalozzi's "mother method" to the teaching of deaf children, as it was being used in the education of hearing children.[a] In this he differed from even the most orally inclined of his predecessors, who still clung to the grammatical method of teaching language.

---

[a] The "mother method," according to Pestalozzi, was the method of acquiring knowledge, as it was used between an infant and his mother, simply by normal, natural, repeated, everyday contact with the things involved in daily living.

The foundations of Hill's teaching principles were these

1.   Deaf children should be taught language in the same way that hearing children learn it, by constant daily use, associated with the proper objects and actions. (As an aid to this, Hill designed a set of charts, each containing sixteen colored pictures, and supplemented by a series of special readers.)

2.   Speech must be the basis of all language, as it is with hearing children. Therefore, oral language must be taught before reading and writing. (His lessons featured simple, but natural, conversations between teacher and child, and between child and child.)

3.   Speech must be used from the beginning as a basis for teaching and communication. (Hill did not exclude the use of natural gestures as a means of understanding, but felt that they could rapidly be replaced by oral language.)

Various German writers of the time supported Hill's views. One of them made these observations:

The teachers of the deaf and dumb are, as a rule, selected from the ordinary school teachers, and must be practical and competent men; the best are those who have already had practical experience in teaching and have acquitted themselves well. The task which they have to perform in a deaf and dumb school is much more difficult and laborious than teaching in an ordinary school. As the subjects of instruction are the same as those taught in an ordinary school, a teacher who intends to devote himself to the instruction of deaf-mutes only requires to master the technicalities of the mechanical portion of their instruction.

In the debates of the Prussian Diet the argument used against the establishment of new deaf and dumb schools was that the teachers of the deaf are so scarce; but this is not a valid reason, as in a very short time a competent school teacher can be transformed into a teacher of the deaf and dumb. In order to induce competent teachers to become instructors of the deaf-mute it is, of course, necessary to offer them pecuniary advantages, as more work is required of them in their new position. (68, p. 161)

Hill was also a master in the training program for teachers. In time he had disciples everywhere in Germany, using his principles in their own varied techniques of teaching. His influence on the German system of teaching the deaf was, no doubt greater than that of any other single person. (8,b, pp. 57-63; 152) He died September 30, 1874, at the age of 69. (108, p. 114)

In England, as more deaf children were brought forward and the need for their education mounted, more asylums were opened and supported by means of charitable subscriptions. In the north of England, the Rev. Fenton of Doncaster determined to open a school for the deaf children of Yorkshire. He went to Paris for advice, and came back full of enthusiasm for the French method.

To arouse interest in raising funds, he had deaf children brought from the school at Manchester to demonstrate at Doncaster. In 1829, the school at Doncaster opened in a rented house, with eleven pupils, under the charge of Charles Baker (1803-1874).

Baker was a native of Birmingham, England, and had served for three years as assistant teacher at the Birmingham Institution under Louis du Puget. As du Puget's disciple he had little use for teaching speech. His committee also preferred the French system, so the school at Doncaster was set up along those lines.

Baker was head of the Doncaster school for forty-five years. During that time he published numerous books to be used as texts in the classrooms. He believed strongly in such devices as the memorization of vocabulary lists, arranged in categories. His *Tables of Genera* listed things "animal, vegetable, and mineral" which the children learned by copying.

His own description of the curriculum at Doncaster listed natural and explanatory signs, dactylology or finger spelling, and writing, taught in that order. Reading appeared to be a corollary to writing. Articulation, he said, should be taught whenever a child had a special aptitude for it, but, in general, he considered it a "specious acquirement."

He advocated beginning by using real objects and teaching the children their names. It was, he said,

a dreary task for beginners to form only letters on fingers and slates,

without usable meaning. Dramatic presentation was used to teach action words.

Grammar was taught by illustrative lessons, rather than by definition. The lessons were arranged in order, according to language principles. The climax was reached in the use of connected language in very short stories. He also advocated encouraging the children to use drawing as a means of expression.

These principles of teaching were incorported in his published textbooks. (139)

In 1819, John Paunceforth Arrowsmith published a book called *The Art of Instructing the Infant Deaf and Dumb*. This book was inspired by his intimate association with his younger brother, who was deaf.

When it was discovered that the child was deaf, his mother determined that it should not rob him of the same opportunities for normal living which she provided for her other children. This included equal discipline in the home, as well as equal privileges.

When he was four, his mother insisted on sending him to school with his older brother, John. The old lady who conducted the school protested that she did not know how to teach him his letters, because he could not hear. His mother retorted that he could see, couldn't he!

The little boy was very quick at imitating and observing the other children. He watched them speak their letters, then turned to the teacher for an explanation. In that way he learned his letters with the other children, using his own lipreading and imitative speech.

The family at home augmented the lessons at school. They spelled out familiar words for the boy with letter blocks, and illustrated them. Because he liked to eat, and also because he was fond of the family cat, they spelled out for him "CAT CAN EAT MEAT," and demonstrated by feeding the cat. Then they muzzled the dog and stated "DOG CANNOT EAT MEAT." In time, they procured a copy of de l'Épée's La Véritable Manière, and added finger spelling and signs to their means of communication with the boy.

The boy was a mischievous little fellow, and often needed to be brought into line at school. Usually the teacher wore a large, checked gingham apron to protect her skirt while she was teaching. One day, for some reason, she came to school in a dainty tea apron instead. The little deaf boy, punished for some mischief in the usual way, was tied to her apron. While her attention was directed elsewhere, an older boy teased the little culprit by pretending to have something exciting in his pocket. Forgetting his restraint, the little boy dashed to look, and tore the dainty apron. Immediately he burst into tears, trying to express to his teacher his sorrow at the damage he had done. But, he added in pantomime, pointing upstairs to her living quarters, if she had worn the big, strong apron, as usual, it would not have torn.

This incident was greeted with tears of joy, when it was related at home, as proof that the boy had normal reasoning power.

In the same way, he was expected to take part with his brothers and sisters in all activities at home. When they said their prayers, he knelt on his father's lap, and did his best to follow by imitation. His voice was described as natural and pleasant.

Because of his experience with his deaf brother, Arrowsmith deplored the English system of herding deaf children into asylums. He felt that the children would do much better to go to their home schools, with their families supplying the extra help they needed at home. Instead of surrounding their methods with secrecy, he advocated that the school masters share their techniques with parents, to enable them to teach their own children. He was convinced that there was no real mystery about teaching deaf children, anyway. His arguments were all the more urgent because, at that time, the institutions were over-crowded and turning children away for lack of room.

Arrowsmith did not believe that the artificial teaching of "utterance" as practiced by the schools was desirable in any way. He found his brother's voice more normal and natural than those of children so taught, and felt it was because he had been allowed to develop imitative speech in his own way, both at home and at school.

Arrowsmith was much impressed by de l'Épée and his methods. His book closed with an English translation of *La Véritable Manière* by de l'Épée. He followed this with a translation of *Surdus Loquens* by Amman, not because he approved of Amman's philosophy, for he did not agree with his emphasis on speech. But de l'Épée includ-ed Amman's work with his own, and since Arrowsmith honored de l'Épée's opinion, he did likewise.

Arrowsmith proposed to publish a textbook for home use in teaching deaf children. It was to be composed mostly of pictures, but arranged in a clear, readable fashion, and not all mixed up, as he considered Watson's to be. Apparently this plan never reached accomplishment. (9)

Mrs. Arrowsmith, the mother of the deaf boy, extended her efforts in behalf of other deaf children. She was a leading member of the committee for the Liverpool School for the Deaf. (75, p. 167)

Among the English exponents of oralism in teaching the deaf, Thomas Arnold held a leading place.

He traced his descent from Robert Arnold, one of three brothers, who, in 1690, went over to Ireland with King William III in his cam-paign against James II. After the war, Robert Arnold received a grant of land in West Cavan. Thomas Arnold's great-grandmother, widowed, became a Moravian, and the family finally settled in Gracehill, a Moravian settlement in Antrim, Ireland. Here his father became a cabinet-maker and married a Scotswoman, and here Thomas was born, April 23, 1816.[a] (167, p. 294)

The young man's literary interests attracted the attention of his pastor, the Rev. George Kirkpatrick, who made him a Sunday School teacher, gave him the run of his library, and offered to finance him if he would enter the University to study for church work. His father could not spare him from the family business at the time, so he remained where he was. Two years later his brother

---

[a] This background clarifies the several contradictions in the literature concerning Ar-nold's national ancestry.

took over the management of the cabinet business, and Arnold became master of the boys' school at Gracehill.

A young deaf man, James Beatty, came to apply for work at the Arnold establishment. Arnold learned signs and fingerspelling in order to talk with him, and was dismayed at the meagerness of expression he found in this form of communication.

He went for a time to work at the Manchester City Mission. In 1840, he applied for a position as assistant teacher at the Yorkshire Institute for the Deaf at Doncaster, under Charles Baker.

When he still found his interest centered in oralism, Baker sent him, in 1841, to study the art of oral teaching under James Rhind, headmaster of the school at Liverpool. He found the use of oralism not at all adequate in this school, because the pupils did not use it among themselves. He tried a class in oral instruction, but there was no place for it on the regular schedule and the pupils resented the extra work involved. Arnold was convinced that a complete separation of the two methods was the only efficient way to teach oralism. However, he had one pupil, George Cochrin, who did so well under oral instruction that Arnold was convinced of its possibilities.

In 1843, he left the schools of the deaf entirely and entered the ministry of the Congregational church. His first parish was the Chapel of Burton-on-Trent. He was married in 1848, and transferred to Smethwick near Birmingham.

Ten year later, finding his wife's health poor and his income inadequate for his needs, he took his family and went to accept a pastorate in Balmain, Sydney, Australia. He had not been there long before the Hon. Thomas Holt, a member of the Legislative Council, heard of his interest in teaching the deaf, and persuaded him to take on the oral education of his deaf son, Frederick.

Within a year and a half, Arnold found it necessary to return to England, taking young Holt with him, and settled in Northampton, where he became pastor, in 1860, of Doddridge Chapel. (167, pp. 294-300)

In 1868, he accepted another deaf pupil, Abraham Farrar, a boy of seven, who had been deafened by scarlet fever at the age of three. He was with Arnold for thirteen years.

He did so well under Arnold's teaching that, in 1881, at the age of twenty, he passed the Cambridge University local examinations, and the London University Matriculation.

> He was the first deaf boy in the United Kingdom to achieve success in a public examination. (75, p. 238)

He qualified as an architect and surveyor, although he never practiced these professions. Instead, he spent his time gathering materials on scholarship for the deaf, including the revision of his teacher's book, *Education of the Deaf*. Farrar died in 1944, at the age of eighty-three. (8,b, p. 76)

After his school began to grow, Arnold resigned his pastorate to give more time to his teaching and writing for the education of the deaf. His first pamphlet *Aures Surdis, The Education of the Deaf and Dumb, A Review of the French and German Systems* was published in 1872. In it he pleaded the cause of oralism with eloquence, supported by practical examples of the advantages of oral language for the deaf as opposed to manual language. He pointed out the difference between a "natural sign," which was a gesture in some pantomimic way descriptive of the idea expressed, and the arbitrary conventional signs invented by de l'Épée. For example, he referred to the use of the thumb to indicate *good* and the little finger to indicate *bad*. This, he declared, was not a sign, but an arbitrary symbol, and went on to say,

> Is he, i.e., the deaf pupil, not in danger from his previous training of imagining some resemblance which does not exist and so of encumbering his reason with a clog instead of a help? (8,a)

Another criticism he made of the French teaching of signs was their adoption of the order of the signs used by the illiterate deaf, considering it a natural order and, therefore, important. Thus the sentence,

> Thomas is whipping his top with a scourge.

became in sign language,

> Thomas top his scourge a with whipping is.

Arnold felt that the teaching of language would be much better served if the normal order of words in a sentence were followed from the beginning.

He also protested what he called "scrap" teaching, in which the pupil was expected to pile up long lists of nouns, adjectives, verbs, etc., before he finally reached the use of sentences. This practice, and the use of the confused word order were, he felt, largely responsible for the "known aversion of the deaf to reading and writing," because they did not feel at home in the language.

This he illustrated with the following analogy:

> Which of our parents, forgetful of nature in his devotion to system, ever thought of arresting this progress and strove to confine us to

breakfasts, dinners, and teas, of nouns, after a time spiced with adjectives, at last, as a special favor, a treat of pronouns and verbs. (8,a)

In support of the German method, he cited the argument that it related the deaf to the language of their environment and gave them the same instrument for thought. Even for those whose lipreading was poor and their speech indistinct, there remained the use of the manual alphabet. They were still able to enjoy reading and writing, since this did no violence to normal language structure. (8,a)

In 1881, Arnold published a more extensive work, *A Method of Teaching the Deaf and Dumb Lipreading and Language.* When the College of Teachers of the Deaf was formed, in 1885, Arnold was requested to provide a manual for them. This book was issued by the College in 1888, under the title *Education of Deaf-Mutes: A Manual for Teachers.*

In 1901, the book was revised and, to some extent, re-written by A. Farrar. He extended the historical section to his own day, as Arnold's original writing had ended with de l'Épée. The sections on anatomy and physiology were brought up to date. But most of the work on teaching language was left largely as Arnold had written it.

The volume was divided into four books. Book One was a brief historical sketch of the history of the deaf. Book Two consisted of definitions and expositions of various methods used in educating the deaf. Book Three was a careful analysis of the Oral System, beginning with a detailed description of sound, and going on to the anatomy and physiology of the speech organs. Book Four gave, in organized detail, instructions for techniques of language teaching in schools for the deaf. Arnold's philosophy was illustrated by this paragraph:

> On the method of teaching grammar there is much room for different opinions. Usually it is applied to language as a set of definitions, illustrated by examples, and to be learned apart from its use as the instrument of thought and intercourse. Nothing can well be more uninteresting or impose a heavier tax on memory. No need to teach it in this manner to the deaf. There is a better way within their reach in the method by which they have learned language. Here the simple sentence is the foundation, consisting as it does of a noun and a verb, which can be taught at first, not by definition, but in their relation as the subject and the action, naming them according to their import. If this is done with a few familiar sentences, the learner will soon find out that *noun,* and its substitute *pronoun,* mean any subject, and *verb* any action or affirmative word. The definition can afterwards be more formally stated when its meaning is made clear by the exercises. (8,b, p. 405)

Arnold's school at Northampton grew into the Northampton High School for the Deaf, and was for eighty years the only institution in Britain for the higher education of the deaf. After the publication of his pamphlets, his work prospered, so that he had to hire an assistant, a young man named Walter Bessant. Arnold was already sixty-seven when he achieved success, but he was eighty-one when he died in 1897.

By this time schools for the deaf were growing up in all countries. In Ireland, the first institution was established in 1816 at Claremont, Glasnevin, near Dublin, with 50 pupils and Joseph Humphrey for its first Master. The opening of this school was due largely to the efforts of a physician of Dublin, Charles Edward Herbert Orpen. He was also the author of a collection of anecdotes and information about the deaf, published in 1836, under the title *Anecdotes and Annals of the Deaf and Dumb.* (8,b, p. 75; 42, Vol. II, p. 313)

The little province of Nova Scotia organized a school for the deaf in Halifax in 1856. James Scott Hutton became its principal after teaching for ten years in the Edinburgh Institute. Hutton did much to advance the education of the deaf in Canada, by means of the textbooks he published for classroom teaching. (8,b, p. 72)

In the northern countries, the most rapid progress was made in Denmark, with a state foundation for schools for the deaf by 1807. Education for deaf children was compulsory by 1840. (39, p. 308; 96)

In Sweden, the first school was the Royal Institute of Stockholm, which opened in 1809, with forty pupils. The queen, herself, presided over the Board of Directors. (42, p. 309)

The Empress Maria Theodorowna took under her protection the Institute at St. Petersburg, Russia, which opened with sixty-one pupils, in 1806. (42, p. 309)

Keller and Ulrich, in the canton of Zürich, Switzerland, used de l'Épée and his methods for their model. They carried on a correspondence with the French teacher for his advice and approval of their work. (42, pp. 127-128)

On the other hand, Naëf, at Yverdon, used strictly oral methods He saw how much his pupils were interested in geography, and so made it one of his major subjects. He was opposed to the teaching of trades in the deaf schools, feeling that this placed the emphasis on the wrong things and detracted from the intellectual development of the pupils. (42, pp. 134-136)

Burki, at the Institution at Bachtelen, near Berne, thought at first that he would follow the Paris system, and even amplify and expand the signs. But he found them too complicated for ordinary teachers and not much use to the pupils after they left school. So he abandoned signs and taught lipreading and imitative speech. (42, pp. 137-140)

As the work with deaf children grew in various countries, it was, naturally, carried to their colonies. In India, it was begun by Haerne in Bombay, in 1884, and in Calcutta by Sinha and Banerji, in 1893. These centers remained mostly shelters and occupational centers until the twentieth century. (75, p. 266)

The nuns from Cabra, Ireland, carried the work to New South Wales in 1875, and also to South Africa in 1863. In the latter place the prejudices of race and religion kept the work from spreading to the native population. By the turn of the century, the education of the colored deaf consisted of three children, taught in a room apart from the white children, in a missionary school at Tuin Plein. (75, p. 266)

The Dutch Reformed Church had a school for deaf children at Worcester, South Africa, in 1881. Gerrit van Asch established one at Christchurch in New Zealand in 1879. (75, p. 266)

William Robson Scott was an English writer who supported the methods of Charles Baker. Trained by Baker, he was, for thirty-six years, principal of the West of England Institution at Exeter. His book *The Deaf and Dumb, their Education and Social Position* appeared in 1870. He advocated using written language as the basic method of teaching, assisted by natural signs. Language, he stated, should be taught by use, not by grammar, combining the colloquial and systematic methods. (8,b, p. 73)

In England, overcrowding in the asylums and their complete isolation from the general educational world was bringing about a serious stagnation in the education of the deaf. Richard Elliott, a teacher of hearing children, accepted a position as assistant teacher at the school for the deaf in the Old Kent Road. He was appalled by what he saw. He stated, as quoted by Hodgson,

> Mr. Thomas James Watson, the headmaster, rarely came into the school. . . . the assistants received no sort of training. . . . not a word of direction, advice, or encouragement was ever given me or indeed to any of us. . . . provided there was an appearance of work it seemed to be the business of no one in particular to see whether it was efficient or otherwise. (75, p. 197)

Joseph Watson's picture dictionary of 1806 was still in use in 1850. There was "a striking engraving of the old watchman with his rattle and lantern," which no longer existed in actual life, while no pictures were found of more recent objects, such as steamboats and railways.

Later Elliott was transferred as senior Master to an extension of the Old Kent Road Asylum which was opened in Margate. Here he had more freedom, and proceeded to prepare the way for reforms by publishing articles concerning the education of the deaf in the *Educational Times*. (75, pp. 198-207)

Susannah Hull, the daughter of a London doctor, became interested in a small girl who was left deaf, blind, and paralyzed by scarlet fever. She studied what she could find of publications on work with handicapped children, both on the Continent and in America. In 1862, she opened a small school in her father's house in St. Mary Abbott's Terrace in Kensington.[a] (40, a, p. 194) The school was planned for children who had speech but had been later deafened by fevers. Her first thought was to preserve the speech of these children. Her efforts were so successful that she soon broadened her work. In six years, the family moved to Warwick Gardens to make more room for the expanding school.

In the Netherlands, the schools for the deaf were still upholding the oral method. One of the most competent and inspiring of these educators was David Hirsch (1813-1895). He was Director of the Rotterdam school for the deaf for thirty-five years, and included the training of teachers in his program.

He was a convinced oralist. Much of his inspiration came from Hill and Jäger in Germany. (104, p. 114) For him, a deaf child's speech had to be so good that the child would use it spontaneously, as a means of communication. His ability and enthusiasm produced results. His teachers went everywhere, carrying his inspiration for the education of the deaf into many places. (75, p. 218)

Two of Hirsch's teachers were instrumental in the revival of oral teaching for the deaf in England. In 1860, Gerrit Van Asch, a young man of twenty-four, was engaged to teach a deaf child in a private family in Manchester. His work was so successful that he was soon able to set up his own school for deaf children in Earl's Court in London.

In 1863, the Baroness Mayer de Rothschild founded a home for Jewish deaf and dumb in Whitechapel. At first the children were taught finger spelling and signs, but Sir Henry Isaacs persuaded the Baroness to investigate oral teaching. His two deaf children had gone to Rotterdam to school, and he was much impressed by the results.

---

[a] DeLand gave the year 1863 for the opening of this school.

So David Hirsch was asked to send another teacher to England. In 1868, William Van Praagh, a young man of twenty-three, came to take charge of the little school in Mount Street. It prospered so quickly that it soon had to move to larger quarters. In four years, under the guidance of Van Praagh, the school was opened to all deaf children, regardless of creed or nationality, in Fitzroy Square, London. It was then placed under the auspices of the Association for the Oral Instruction of the Deaf and Dumb, which also opened a training school for teachers at the same place. This was the first college for teachers of the deaf in the English-speaking world.

At about the same time, a Mr. and Mrs. St. John Ackers of Huntley Manor, near Gloucester, became interested in the education of the deaf, for the most poignant of reasons, because their little daughter was deaf. Finding so much disagreement among the authorities as to the best method, they toured the schools of Europe and America to see for themselves what could be done for their child. When they returned to England, they decided in favor of oral instruction, and sent a young teacher, Arthur Kinsey, to Germany for training. By 1877, a Society was formed *For Training Teachers of the Deaf and the Diffusion of the German System*. In 1878, the training college was opened in Ealing, under Kinsey's direction.

To all this progress, the established asylums for the deaf remained obstinately opposed, except for Richard Elliott at Margate. He visited other English institutions for the deaf in an effort to foster some reform. At Doncaster, he found James Howard who had succeeded Charles Baker, attempting to teach some speech. With Howard, he planned a conference of principals of schools for the deaf, to be held on the premises of the Social Service Association.

Thomas Watson was invited to this metting, but he did not come. The Committee of the Asylum of Old Kent Road passed a resolution stating that Elliott's participation in the meeting was "very distasteful." But many others came, including the principals of the new oral schools. They added their voices to those of Elliott and Howard in favor of reform in schools for the deaf. The whole meeting was persuaded to visit the nearby Schoentheil school to see what skillful oral teaching could do.

The next year Watson resigned, and Elliott was appointed head of the Old Kent Road Asylum, as well as of the Margate branch. The resolution disapproving his participation in the conference of principals was rescinded. Oral teaching of the deaf was again on its way in England. (81, pp. 233-235)

In Groningen, Netherlands, Charles Guyot was carrying on the school his father had founded. He was much taken up with the physical development of his pupils, which he felt their families neglected. He was also impressed with the various attempts at medical treatment for deafness. In 1827, he assisted while eighty-one of his deaf-mute pupils had their eardrums pierced in an effort to improve their hearing (26; 29, pp. 7-9)

He made a serious effort to secure the benefits of education for all deaf children within his reach. To accomplish this he set up the principle that all deaf and dumb children were to be equally welcome at his school, no matter who or what their parents were; children from Groningen were to receive no special privileges over any others. Guyot was instrumental in the writing of a law that required all children born deaf to be reported to the educational department of the village or city in which they resided. If they did not live under the jurisdiction of any department, the parents were permitted to correspond directly with Guyot concerning their child. (66)

Arnoldus Wilhelm Alings, who became head of the administration at Groningen, November 1, 1854, was much attracted by the German method. He traveled to see the best schools, mostly in Germany. At first he continued with the methods of the Guyots, but gradually became more and more influenced by the German method.

After he became Director of Instruction, he rearranged the classes to group the children according to their language ability rather than their age. He hammered at his teachers to keep the children talking. Always when he entered a classroom, he complained, he heard only the instructor's voice, not the children. And he felt that a language is learned not so much by hearing as by speaking it.

At the age of seventy, after thirty-seven years of work for the school, he asked to be released. Three years later, he died, in Utrecht.

In France, the system of teaching methodical signs was gradually weakening in favor of more attention to verbal language by means of writing. Jean Jacques Valade-Gabel, born September 23, 1801, in Sarlat, was a teacher at the Paris Institute for Deaf-Mutes from October 9, 1825 until July 25, 1838. In 1839, he was named Director of the school at Bordeaux. Having been a student of Pestalozzi, he tried to use the "mother method" of teaching language by means of writing. Speech was soon added in the school at Bordeaux, as well as in a number of other schools in France. Finally, when he became Inspector-General of the Institutions for the Deaf in France, he tried to introduce Pestalozzi's "mother method" of teaching language by use in all the schools. He had little immediate response from the teachers. (60; 91) But his work received the approval of the Institute of Paris. In 1857, he published a description of his methods under the title, *Methode a la portes des instituteurs primaires, pour enseigner aux sourds-muets la langue Francaise sans l'intermediare de langue des signes.*[a]

Although the results of his efforts fell short of what he hoped to achieve, the work of Valade-Gabel did much to loosen the hold of the sign language in the schools of France. His successor, M. Claveau (1826-1904), spent the first year of his office visiting schools for the deaf in neighboring countries. What he saw influenced him favorably toward oral instruction.

Valade-Gabel's philosophy was introduced into the United States at the New York Institute for the Deaf in 1830, by his associate, M. Leon Vaïsse. At that time, methodical signs were the accepted technique of teaching in the New York Institute brought from Hartford by the Principal, Harvey Prindle Peet. After four years of work by Vaïsse, they were still not entirely eradicated, although the trend was toward more natural methods of teaching. (8,b, pp. 50-51; 60; 75, pp. 261-262)

Meanwhile, schools for the deaf in the United States spread rapidly from one state to another. Some were begun as small private schools, and later taken over by the public school system. Many had been instituted as benevolent asylums and were given state support, with the addition of more educational features. Very many were created as state schools from the beginning. These were all residential schools, and followed the manual system of education established by Gallaudet at Hartford.

Outside the institutions, there was not the same universal satisfaction with their methods.

Horace Mann (1796-1859), was a believer in a state school system. In 1837, he became secretary of the first Massachusetts school board. Two years later, he brought about the opening of the first American Teacher's Training College, at Lexington.

He was also interested in the education of handicapped children, and, through his association with Seguin, aroused American interest in their welfare. He did not approve of education by signs for deaf children, and tried to foster interest in oral education for them.

He was joined in this interest by Samuel Gridley Howe (1801-1876), the Director of the Massachusetts School for the Blind. Howe taught Laura Bridgeman, a deaf-blind child, by means of the

---

[a] Method for primary instructors of teaching the French language to deaf mutes without the intermediary of the language of signs.

manual alphabet, and regretted later that he had not tried to teach her speech.

In 1843, Mann and Howe made a trip to Europe to visit the schools for the deaf on the Continent. In the German schools, they were amazed to see how well deaf children were using lipreading and speech. They returned to America, full of enthusiasm for the oral method. Mann published a report, advocating the use of the oral system in America. This awakened the interest of a number of parents, who began to demand speech for their deaf children.

In 1844, G. E. Day of the New York Institution, and Lewis Weld of the American School, also made a trip to Europe to tour the deaf schools. But they were not impressed with what they saw, and came back satisfied with their own methods. In 1851, Harvey Prindle Peet, who had been Gallaudet's assistant at Hartford, and was now Principal of the New York Institution, made the same tour. He also was unimpressed with the oral method.

Day reported that,

> in spite of the peculiar difficulties, even a deaf-mute from birth, by unwearied pains and the expenditure of much time, might to a certain extent be taught to articulate in English, I have no doubt.

If parents have the leisure, he would not dissuade them from the attempt, he said, but felt it would not be practical "as a regular part of a system of education." (60, p. XXVI)

In 1859, Day made a second trip to Europe. On his return, he said that he

> variously estimated at from 1/5 to 1/10 of the whole number consisting of semi-mutes and mutes who became deaf after having once learned to speak, and now and then those who possess special aptitude, mentally and physically, for this kind of work, may be taught with more or less advantage to articulate mechanically and to read upon the lips. (168, p. XXVII)

Near Boston, forces were gathering to promote the teaching of oral education to the deaf. These forces centered around three small girls, all unknown to one another at the time.

One of them was Mabel Hubbard, the daughter of Gardiner Green Hubbard, deafened by scarlet fever when she was almost four. Her mother did everything she could to preserve her speech. Mary True, a teacher of hearing children, was engaged as governess. She used lipreading entirely in talking to Mabel, and tried to find ways to improve the little girl's articulation.

Another of the three was Jeanie Lippitt, the daughter of the

Governor of Rhode Island. She, also, lost her hearing from scarlet fever at the age of three. Her mother undertook to teach her, herself, guided by Samuel Howe, who had never given up his interest in the oral teaching of deaf children.

The third of the small girls was Fanny Cushing, who became deaf at three and a half. She was placed in the care of Harriet Rogers, a teacher of hearing children, whose sister had been one of the teachers of Laura Bridgeman. Rogers received her information on teaching articulation from a newspaper clipping about the German method. With this, and some assistance from Howe, she taught Fanny speech. At first she used finger spelling also, but after she met the Lippits and saw how well Jeanie could lipread, she dropped all manual communication and used lipreading with Fanny. (43,a,b; 60)

Soon these families all joined forces to encourage the same type of teaching for other deaf children. On March 16, 1864, Howe, Hubbard, and other interested men, petitioned the Massachusetts General Court for an act to incorporate an oral school for the deaf in the state. It was defeated through the influence of the school at Hartford. (43,a, pp. 32-33)

Hubbard then persuaded Rogers to open a private school in Chelmsford, Massachusetts. He gave the school his support in every way, including financial assistance. For, though it had eight pupils in 1867, only two were paying full tuition. But the school served as an advertisement to the public, entertaining many visitors to show the things its pupils accomplished through oral education.

In 1866, Hubbard again prepared a petition for the Massachusetts legislature, appealing for an oral school. He demonstrated the little group from the Chelmsford school before committees. The American School also sent children from Hartford, to show their learning in manual language. Again the influence of the Hartford school was too strong, and the bill faced defeat.

Governor Bullock had been sympathetic, so Hubbard appealed directly to him. By coincidence, that same day, the Governor had received a letter from a philanthropist who offered to donate $50,000 towards the establishment of an oral school for the deaf, at Northampton, Massachusetts. This man was John Clarke. He became interested in the problem of deafness because he was gradually losing his own hearing.

The Governor sent a message to the legislature, urging the establishment of an oral school, under state jurisdiction, Mrs. Josiah Quincy opened her house in Boston for a demonstration. She invited youngsters from the Chelmsford school, and their teacher.

On March 16, 1867, a number of legislators and reporters came to see for themselves. When they saw Jeanie Lippit, now fifteen, and Roscoe Green, eighteen, both deaf but chatting away with each other about their teen-age affairs, "their skepticism melted away."

Harriet Rogers and her pupils were moved to Northampton, to organize the Clarke School for the Deaf in October, 1867. (36)

A member of the Boston School Board, a man named Dexter King, attended all the hearings of the Massachusetts legislature that led to the establishment of the Clarke School. Immediately, he began to agitate for a branch of the Clarke School to be opened in Boston. This did not prove practical, but in 1869, an oral day school was opened instead, with Sarah Fuller as principal and Mary True as assistant. The school was first known as the Boston School for Deaf-Mutes, but in 1877 the name was changed to the Horace Mann School.

A few months before the opening of Clarke School, a small Jewish oral school was opened in New York by Bernard Engelman. A few years later it was recognized and given support by the state of New York. It then became a non-sectarian school, and was called the New York Institution for the Improved Instruction of Deaf-Mutes. (8,b, p. 97; 75, p. 283)

Alexander Graham Bell was born March 3, 1847, in the family home at South Charlotte Street, Edinburgh, Scotland.[a] (92, p. 18) He was the second son of Alexander Melville Bell, who was the second son of Alexander Bell. Born on his grandfather's birthday, he was named in his honor, and was always called "Aleck" by his family. The name "Graham" he added at the age of eleven because of his fondness for a friend of his father, whose name was Alexander Graham. He later used this middle name to distinguish himself from his father and grandfather.

His grandfather, Alexander Bell, began making his living as a shoemaker. Later he became an actor in the Theatre Royal in Edinburgh, then returned to his home town of St. Andrews and taught English diction. Still later, he moved to London. (92, p. 15-19)

Alexander Melville Bell followed the family tradition of teaching diction and elocution. He was very much interested in the general subject of speech and language. He had dreams of fostering the adoption of a universal language, which could serve as a common denominator for all languages. For this purpose he invented a

---

[a] DeLand placed the event at 93 Hope St., Edinburgh, and said that the family lived at a later time at 13 S. Charlotte Street. (43,a, p. 193)

system which he called Visible Speech.[b] These symbols were designed as a pictorial abbreviation of the fundamental positions of the speech organs in giving utterance to the sounds.

The diagram and passage on pages 144, 145 and 146 illustrate the principle of the method.

The symbols have the same value in all languages. Consequently, when the meaning of the symbols is known, the sounds of the language may be deduced with certainty from their Visible Speech writing.

The explanations are FOR THE TEACHER ONLY. The learner need not know the theory of the system. (19, pp. vi-viii)

In spite of its ingenuity, and the eloquence of its inventor, the system had only a temporary vogue, and was forgotten in a relatively short time.

The Bell family had three sons, and they were a close-knit family. The mother was extremely hard of hearing, from the age of four, following an attack of scarlet fever. When she recovered from the fever and asked why the birds no longer sang, her parents realized how deaf she was, and engaged a governess to help her keep her speech. No one seemed to have thought of lipreading. She used speech normally, all her life, but to gather what people said to her, she used an ear trumpet and the manual alphabet. It was not surprising that her son, in his later work with deaf children, needed to be convinced that lipreading was as practical as speech, for the deaf. (43,b, pp. 115-117; 92, p. 61)

In 1867, the youngest of the three sons died of tuberculosis. A year later, at the death of the grandfather, Alexander Bell, the family moved to London and took over some of his clients in elocution.

Here Alexander Graham Bell came in contact with Susannah Hull and her little oral school for deaf children in Warwick Gardens. She was interested in the apparent possibilities of the Visible Speech symbols in teaching speech to the deaf. Bell arranged to work with her, attempting to adapt the symbols for such use. For a while their enthusiasm was great. But the method was soon found impractical and gradually abandoned. (43,b, pp. 115-117)

In 1870, the oldest Bell son succumbed to tuberculosis. A medical examination confirmed the dread suspicion that the one son remaining was suffering from the same disease. Anxiously, the family cast about for some way to save him. They hoped a better climate might help, and moved to Brantford, in Ontario, Canada, the same

[b] This term, at this place in history, does not refer to the Visible Speech mechanism which is an electronic device more recently developed by the Bell Telephone Laboratories.

Visible Speech

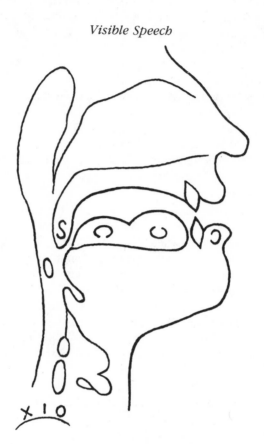

Fundamental Symbols

C Back of Tongue   S Nasal passage open

O Top   "   "   X Glottis closed

U Point "   "   I   "   vocalizing

Ɔ Lips   O   "   open (aspirate)

(throat aspirate (whisper)

Explanatory Preface

Those who are not acquainted with the principles of Visible Speech might, with a little observation, discover the basis of the system for themselves, from the writing of familiar words. Nevertheless, a little explanation is a great assistance. The following are the fundamental points:

A curved line means a consonant.
A straight line means a vowel.
A line within a curve means a vocal consonant.

Consonants

The direction of the curve denotes:

To left, (**C**) formation by back of tongue.

To right, (**Ɔ**) ” ” lips.

Convex above, (**∩**) ” ” tip of tongue.

Concave ” , (**◡**) ” ” point of tongue.

The varieties of curves denote:

Primary, (**C**) central emission of breath.

Divided, (**Ɜ**) side ” ” ”

Mixed, (**Ƈ**) central emission ⎰ with modification by

Mixed, divided, (**Ɛ**) side emission ⎱ two parts of the mouth.

Shut, (**ᑯ**) oral stoppage of breath.

Nasal, (**Ƈ̧**) oral stoppage of breath with emission
through the nose.

Vowels

A point, or a hook, on a straight line denotes the vowel positions of the tongue. Thus:

On left side of line,   (⌐) back of mouth.

On right   ”   ”   ” , (⌐) front ”   ”

On both sides”   ” , (⌐) mixed, back and front.

At top   ”   ” , (⌐) high.

At bottom   ”   ” , (⌐) low.

At both ends   ”   ” , (⌐) mid elevation.

A cross bar on a line denotes rounding or contraction of the lips.
   Thus: ⌐ ⌐ ⌐

Readings

2. ꝋꞹꝏꝐ

Ɪꞹ ꝓꞹꝍꞮꞩ ꞷꞮꝩꞷ ꞹꞮ ꝍꞮꞢꝏꞹ
Ɪꞹꝍ ꝺꞮꞹꞮꞩꞹ Ɪꝍ ꞹꞮ ꝍꞮꝏꞹꞹ, ꞹꝓ
Ɪꞹ ꝓꞹꝍꞮꝐ ꞷꞮꞹꞮꝩꝍ ꝩꞷꝓꝐ ꝓꞷ
ꝍꞮꞢ Ɪꝍꞷ ꝑꞷꞮꞹꞮꝩꝩꝍ ꝑꞮꞢ Ɪ ꞷꝓꞢꞮ
ꞹꝓꞷ.   (19, p. 66)

Key to Readings

2. WISDOM

As water leaves the heights and gathers in the depths, so is wisdom received from on high and preserved by a lowly soul.

                                     Talmud (19, p. 73)

year. (92, pp. 40-45)

The year previous to this move, Alexander Melville Bell had given a series of lectures at the Lowell Institute in Boston, Massachusetts, on Visible Speech and elocution. He now returned to Boston for another series of lecture engagements.

Sarah Fuller had attended the first lecture series and was much impressed by them. When she heard of Bell's return, she wrote to him, requesting that he visit her school for deaf children, and train her teachers in Visible Speech. He replied that his classes in Ontario demanded his return, but suggested his son, Alexander Graham Bell, as a substitute.

In April 1871, Alexander Graham Bell came to Sarah Fuller's school. The school committee was persuaded to appropriate $500 for his services.

It was at this school that Bell saw, with astonishment, how readily the children used lipreading for communication. From then on, he was a convinced supporter of lipreading as well as speech, in the education of deaf children.

Bell spent two months at the school in Boston. Then he was invited to the Clarke School at Northampton, and also spent several weeks at the American school at Hartford. Again enthusiasm ran high for the Visible Speech method, for a time. But again it proved unwieldy and impractical for little children, giving them an additional translation to master on their way to articulate speech. Gradually the device was abandoned. But the efforts at teaching speech stimulated by Bell and his associates developed a nucleus of teachers who were strong advocates for the oral method of teaching the deaf in the United States. (43,a, 195-198; b, 115-117; 92, pp. 49-51)

In 1872, Bell opened a training school for teachers of the deaf in Boston. His plan was to make it an oral training school, using Visible Speech as one fundamental technique. The opposition of the big deaf schools, with their silent methods, soon made this impossible, so he returned to the traditional family profession, and made it a School of Vocal Physiology or Elocution. (43,a, p. 209; 92, pp. 55-56)

Mabel Hubbard, the litte deaf girl who had helped to start oralism in the United States, was now grown to young womanhood. She spent six months in Germany, to perfect her use of lipreading. Recently returned home, she came to Bell's school in Boston for further improvement of her speech. It was not long until the young teacher fell in love with his student. After this, he was a frequent visitor at the Hubbard home on Brattle Street, in Cambridge. While at the Sarah Fuller school in Boston, Bell had been inspired to find some mechanical means of making speech visible. For a while, he tried a manometric flame.[a] Then he began to experiment with the electrical transmission of sound, in an attempt to develop amplification. It was these experiments which finally led to the invention of the telephone.

In the winter of 1872-1873, while he was dividing his time between his elocution classes and electrical experiments, Bell lived in a rooming house at 35 West Newton Street. A little deaf boy of five from Haverhill, Massachusetts, named George Sanders, was brought to him at this place. His father wanted the child to have speech training from Bell, and had him live with a nurse at the same rooming house, so that Bell could teach him outside of his own working hours.

Bell spent his summer vacation at his family's home in Ontario. When he returned to Boston in the fall of 1873, it was decided that little George would be happier in his grandmother's home in Salem. Bell moved there also, and made the hour-long trip to Boston and back daily by train.

His hostess was very indulgent with the young inventor. She allowed him to use the basement and finally the whole top floor of the house for his experiments. For three years, he worked in this fashion.

> All of this time, Bell was giving his lectures at Boston University, maintaining his classroom in Beacon Street, and going back nightly to the Sanders house in Salem, where an eager little boy flattened his small nose against a window-pane, watching for the tall figure hurrying up the street. (92, p. 69)

Until the child's bedtime, Bell's time apparently belonged to little George. He taught him speech, but not lipreading. In order to tell him stories about the things he had seen during the day, Bell made a glove on which he printed letters, and by pointing to these in some way communicated his tales to the child.

After George had gone to bed, Bell spent long hours at his experiments. Mrs. Sanders used to cut his candles shorter than usual, so that when they burned out, he would be forced to go to bed. Sanders, the father of his pupil, and Hubbard, the father of the

---

[a]A manometric flame was a gas flame whose height was changed by changing the pressure of the gas by means of sound waves directed against a diaphragm. When this changing flame was seen in a series of rotating mirrors, the resultant visual image made a pattern consistent with the pressure patterns of the sound waves impinging upon the diaphragm.

girl he loved, gave him the financial support to carry on with his experiments.

On his twenty-ninth birthday, Bell was granted the patent on the telephone. The Hubbard family finally withdrew their opposition to their daughter's marriage to an impoverished young inventor. Alexander Graham Bell and Mabel Hubbard were married July 11, 1877. (92, pp. 114-183)

One of the prizes Bell received for his work with electricity was the Allessandro Volta Prize, named in memory of the father of electricity. With $200,000 of this money he founded The Volta Bureau, in 1887, "for the increase and diffusion of knowledge relating to the deaf."

In 1890, there was founded the American Association for Teaching Speech to the Deaf, largely through Bell's efforts. This developed into a national organization of teachers and educators interested in oral instruction for the deaf.

Bell was much disturbed about the scarcity of proper speech teaching for deaf children in America. He cited instances, such as that of a boy who lost his hearing at the age of twelve. He was sent to a school for the deaf, and when he graduated he had lost his speech entirely. He found hard-of-hearing children in these schools, who could hear the voice of the speaker, but needed help in understanding. Nothing was done to utilize this hearing, and these children had no speech.

Bell made a statistical study of deafness, and showed that the isolation of the deaf within a sign language of their own was forcing constant intermarriage and increasing the proportionate rate of hereditary deafness. He advocated that deaf children should be educated orally and in day school situations, where they could maintain normal social contacts. He improved the United States census forms in 1890, so that the deaf could more accurately be counted in the total population. It was due to Bell that the term "deaf" was officially substituted for "deaf-mute."

Bell was one of the first to advocate that deaf children begin their learning of speech by imitation of whole words, with meaning. This was in opposition to the long-used element method, in which separate speech elements were taught first, then combined into meaningless syllables, before the child acquired speech words for communication. Under Bell's method, children were to be taught to understand whole words and sentences in lipreading and writing, and then to imitate the speech for them. Pronunciation was to be corrected as the child used the speech thus acquired. (8,b, p. 100; 92, pp. 246-254)

Bell lived to be seventy-five years old, to enjoy the successes of many of his ventures, and to continue his varied interests in future developments through the young men of science with whom he was constantly surrounded. He died August 2, 1922, at his home in Cape Breton. (92, p. 363)

Out of the controversy concerning the silent and oral methods of teaching the deaf came a compromise that has been typically American. A number of the schools adopted what they called the combined method, which was intended to make use of the best in both approaches to teaching the deaf. This compromise received the support of the Gallaudet family.

The various schools made their own decisions as to their interpretation of what a combined method should include. They taught articulation, lipreading, manual spelling, signs, reading, and writing in various proportions and at various age levels, in what seemed to them the most practical means of giving education and communication skills to the deaf children under their charge.

In 1856, Amos Kendall, wanting to found a small private school for the deaf in Washington, D.C., made contact with the Gallaudets, Edward Miner Gallaudet, the younger son of Thomas Hopkins Gallaudet, expressed interest in the project and was given charge of the new school, which was called Kendall School. After seven years, Congress refounded the school as Columbia Institution, with Edward Miner Gallaudet for its president. In 1894 the preparatory department was named Kendall School, to retain the name of the original founder. The Institution was renamed Gallaudet College, in honor of Thomas Hopkins Gallaudet.

This college became, in 1864, the first and only institution of higher learning in the world exclusively for the deaf. In 1891, a teachers' training department was added.

When Edward Miner Gallaudet heard of the work of the Clarke School in oral teaching, he went to see for himself how the method worked. Then he took a tour to Europe, in 1867, to visit the schools in other countries. He returned, still satisfied with the silent method, but felt that the whole matter should receive public consideration.

In 1868, he called a conference of representatives from the schools for the deaf in the United States to meet in Washington, D.C. The principals of fifteen of the twenty-five schools then in existence came to the conference in May of that year. After five days of discussion, the conference unanimously adopted this resolution:

In the opinion of this Conference, it is the duty of all institutions for the deaf and dumb to provide adequate means of imparting instruction in articulating and lip reading to such of their pupils as may be able to profit in exercises of this nature. (8,b, pp. 97-98)

This, again, left the decision of the type of method to be used entirely to the individual schools.

In Spain, the cradle of the art, there was an interval of nearly two centuries before it was revived. D. Jh. Miguel d'Alea, a pupil of de l'Épée, founded a school in Madrid early in the nineteenth century, and followed the French method exclusively. (39, pp. 211-213)

His successor, D. Tiburgio Hernandez, directed the school in Madrid after 1814. He took the opposite direction and sought to revive the original Spanish method of teaching. He studied what he could find of descriptions of the work of Pedro de Ponce de Leon and Bonet. He differed from Bonet in attaching more importance to the use of the manual alphabet, and to the teaching of lipreading. His technique for both lipreading and speech was to have the teacher sit facing the pupil and speak slowly, having him watch the formation of each sound. He absolutely forbade the use of the leather thong, the fingers, or any other object in the pupil's mouth, to shape the speech organs. His method was rigidly analytic, with the sounds taught one by one, then combined into syllables, and finally, words. (42, pp. 219-227)

In Italy, meanwhile, work in teaching the deaf had proceeded along much the same lines as it had in other countries. After the school at Rome was founded by the Abba Silvestri, other schools for the deaf were established in various Italian cities.

Tomaso Pendola (1800-1883) founded the school at Sienna, and remained as its director for fifty years. He followed a modified form of the French system, at first, but soon became enthusiastic about the possibilities of oral teaching. His support of oralism did much to encourage its introduction into Italian schools.

The Abba Serafino Balestra (1834-1886) was in charge of the school at Como. He was trained as a manual teacher, but he, too, became interested in the possibilities of speech for the deaf. In 1867, he went to Rotterdam to see the work of David Hirsch. What he saw convinced him of the value of oralism. He went back to Italy, where he did all he could to spread oral teaching of the deaf in his own country.

Eventually, he went to South America, to Buenos Aires. There he opened the first school for the deaf on that continent. He remained with it until his death in 1886. (8,b, p. 103; 75, pp. 241-242)

The most prominent leader of the "pure oral method" in Italy was the Abba Guilio Tarra (1832-1889). He was a native of Milan, and entered the church for the purpose of preparing himself for mission work. In 1854, Count Paul Taverna founded the Institution for the Indigent Deaf at Milan. The Abba Tarra was persuaded to become its director.

He entered his new work with his characteristic enthusiasm. At first he taught by the French method. Gradually, he abandoned the sign approach to language, and used objects and actions directly in connection with writing and manual spelling. Speech and lipreading were soon included, wherever they seemed practical.

Not satisfied with his results, the Abba Tarra decided that the use of too many methods was a disadvantage. He also felt that his pupils' dependence on manual spelling and writing for communication prevented them from feeling at home in speech as a living language. So he made all other methods secondary to speech teaching, and abandoned manualism entirely. He stated,

> It is on these grounds that the method we follow is called pure oral perceptive: oral, because the teaching is given by speech alone, articulated and read on the lips; perceptive, because speech is taught in the presence of the fact immediately perceived, or recalled to the sense and intelligence by means of known words; pure, because it is unmixed, and is neither preceded nor followed by means capable of attenuating or confusing the efficacy of living speech. (8,b, p. 105; 128, pp. 9-14)

The growing enthusiasm for oralism in teaching the deaf brought about the desire of the teachers to meet and discuss their various methods and problems. The first International Conference of Teachers of the Deaf was called in Paris in 1878. Plans had not been organized well enough in advance, so it was international in little more than name. However, plans were there made to hold a real international conference, two years later at Milan. (8,b, pp. 103-105; 75, pp. 242-243)

On September 6, 1880, educators of the deaf from all countries which then had such schools, assembled at Milan for an International Congress. The Abba Tarra was its president.

The Congress commenced its initial sitting on Monday, 6th September, at Twelve, noon. (192, p. 9)

An inaugural address was delivered. The rules and regulations of the Congress were read, and election of officers was held by ballot. "After considerable delay," the results were announced. They included a general president and secretary, and a vice-president and vice-secretary from each of five countries, Italy, Germany, France and "the English-speaking section," which shared the honors between England and the United States. The meeting was then adjourned until the next day at 9 A.M. (192, pp 9-11)

The next morning, the Congress began the discussions. The members decided to pass over the first two questions posed by the preceding conference in Paris, on "School Buildings" and "Teaching," and to proceed at once to Section III, on "Methods."

Among the proceedings of that day were a paper by Mrs. B. St. John Ackers, read in French, relating the exhaustive inquiries made by herself and her husband as to the best method of instruction for their little deaf daughter, and their conclusion that the "German" system was best.

M. L'Abbé de la Place, of Soissons, mentioned that the schools in France now use all methods.

Dr. Edward Miner Gallaudet, President of the Deaf-Mute College, Washington, D.C., read a paper in French, defending the "combined " system, and maintained that signs were the natural language of the deaf, as also the mother language of all mankind.

The Reverend Thomas Arnold, Private School, Northampton, England, read a paper in favor of the "articulating system." He had twenty years experience with that system and was of the opinion that it placed the deaf on the same platform that we ourselves occupy.

The Reverend Thomas Gallaudet, Rector of St. Ann's Church for Deaf-Mutes, New York, replied. Having used the sign language for fifty years, he believed fully in its importance to the deaf-mute, and that it was necessary in order to lift him up from ignorance to ideas.

Padre Marchio of Sienna exclaimed, simply, in English, "Come and hear our pupils."

A resumé of a paper by Mr. Richard Elliott, Headmaster of the Asylum for the Deaf and Dumb, London and Margate, was given in French by M. Leon Vaïsse. Mr. Elliott was of the opinion that experience teaches the "Combined" system to be the best.

M. L'Abbé Balestra, Director of the Institution at Como, replied that experience in Italy had shown the pure oral method to be the best.

Miss Hull, Private School, Kensington, England, read her paper in French, upon her varied experience in teaching the deaf.

The President proposed to close the sitting with a resolution. After a long and animated discussion, Dr. Peet, New York, proposed that the resolution be referred to a committee for formulation. This was put to a motion and lost. The resolution, as put to the meeting, was as follows:

I

The Congress—
Considering the incontestable superiority of speech over signs in restoring the deaf-mute to society, and in giving him a more perfect knowledge of language.
Declares—
That the oral method ought to be preferred to that of signs for the education and instruction of the deaf and dumb.

The Resolution was carried almost unanimously, the members in its favor being about 160, as nearly as could be ascertained; and the dissentients 4. The result was greeted with loud applause, and the meeting then adjourned.[a] (192, pp. 16-20)

In the following days of the Congress, these resolutions were adopted:

II

The Congress—
Considering that the simultaneous use of speech and signs has the disadvantage of injuring speech, lipreading and precision of ideas,
Declares—
That the Pure Oral Method ought to be preferred.

III

The Congress—
Considering that a great number of the deaf and dumb are not receiving the benefit of instruction, and that this condition is owing to the "impotence" (impotenza) of families and of institutions,
Recommends—
That Governments should take the necessary steps that all the deaf and dumb may be educated.

IV

The Congress—
Considering that the teaching of the speaking-deaf by the Pure Oral Method should resemble as much as possible that of those who hear and speak—
Declares—
1. That the most natural and effective means by which the speaking-deaf may acquire the knowledge of language is the "intuitive" method, viz., that which consists in setting forth, first by speech, and then by writing, the objects and the facts which are placed before the eyes of the pupils.
2. That in the first, or maternal, period the deaf-mute ought to be led to the observation of grammatical forms by means of examples and of

---

[a] "This was carried by 116 votes to 16." (75, p. 243)

practical exercises, and that in the second period he ought to be assisted to deduce from these examples the grammatical rules expressed with the utmost simplicity and clearness.

3. That books written with words and in the forms of language known to the pupil, can be put into his hands at anytime.

V

The Congress—

Considering the want of books sufficiently elementary to help the gradual and progressive development of language,

Recommends—

That the teachers of the Oral System should apply themselves to the publication of special works on the subject.

VI

The Congress—

Considering the results obtained by the numerous inquiries made concerning the deaf and dumb of every age and every condition long after they had quitted school, who, when interrogated upon various subjects, have answered correctly, with a sufficient clearness of articulation, and read the lips of their questioners with the greatest facility.

Declares—

1. That the deaf and dumb taught by the Pure Oral Method do not forget after leaving school the knowledge which they have acquired there, but develop it further by conversation and reading, which have been made so easy for them.

2. That in their conversation with speaking persons they make use exclusively of speech.

3. That speech and lipreading, so far from being lost, are developed by practice.

VII

The Congress—

Considering that the education of the deaf and dumb by speech has peculiar requirements; considering also that the experience of teachers of deaf-mutes is almost unanimous,

Declares—

1. That the most favourable age for admitting a deaf child into a school is from eight to ten years.

2. That the school term ought to be seven years at least; but eight years would be preferable.

3. That no teacher can effectually teach a class of more than ten children in the Pure Oral Method.

VIII

The Congress—

Considering that the application of the Pure Oral Method in institutions where it is not yet in active operation, should be—to avoid the certainty of failure—prudent, gradual, progressive,

Recommends—

1. That the pupils newly received into the schools should form a class by themselves, where instruction should be given in speech.

2. That these pupils should be absolutely separated from others too far advanced to be instructed by speech and whose education will be completed by signs.

3. That each year a new speaking class be established, until all older pupils taught by signs have completed their education. (192, pp. 5-8)

Section 3 of Resolution 7 is particularly noteworthy, in that it was made at a time when sixty children was considered a good class for one teacher to handle in the hearing schools. (75, p. 243)

Most of the educators who attended the Conference at Milan went home fired by renewed fervor to inspire progress in the education of the deaf. The oral method was adopted as the preferred method in all countries except the United States.

Governments everywhere undertook the responsibility of supporting and supervising the education of the deaf. Finland, in particular, early worked out a system of placing their small deaf children in foster homes near the schools, so that they need not be herded into large institutions.

From this time on the education of the deaf held a recognized place in the responsible world of educational progress.

As the nineteenth century advanced, educators in all countries shifted their focus of attention more and more from the subject matter to the child. In the teaching of the deaf, this consideration of the environmental and developmental needs of children stimulated renewed interest in their need for oral language. Wherever earnest and dedicated teachers set their minds to the task of oral instruction for deaf children, their pupils responded with successful use of speech, lipreading, and language.

Opposition to the oral method was great from the advocates of the silent method. In some instances, this opposition was largely inertia, and fear of the enormity of the task in large, overcrowded schools. In some, it was a sincere belief in the silent method, as the traditional and, therefore, the best method of teaching the deaf.

The United States was the only real stronghold for the silent method, after the Conference at Milan. Other countries made earnest efforts to incorporate the recommendations of the Congress into their schools. In the United States, also, instruction in oralism began to spread more and more rapidly, growing by its own success, side by side with the existing manual methods.

Chapter 9

Breaking the Barrier
of Silence

In the twentieth century, the physical sciences came for the first time in a significant way to the aid of the humanistic approach to the problems of the deaf. Whole realms were opened up by the discovery that more useful residual hearing remained in most cases than had been suspected, and electronics made it possible to exploit this residual hearing in ways hitherto undreamed-of.

As we have traced the history of the deaf up to the twentieth century, we have seen the gradual development of better techniques for education and greater public responsibility for training. Now a new attack was made on the handicap itself that was to prove revolutionary in breaking through the barrier of silence.

Earlier diagnosis and scientific improvements in the instruments for testing hearing brought to light the fact that in most cases more hearing remained to the individual than had been suspected in past times. The development of electronic amplification of sound made usable this residual hearing to a degree never before dreamed possible.

During the closing years of the nineteenth century, the tendency was still to follow old patterns. In the United States, particularly, there were in use a variety of teaching methods and, more frequently, a deliberate combination of methods. The "Rochester Experiment," fostered by Z. F. Westervelt, at the Rochester School in New York, in 1878, was a simultaneous use of finger-spelling, with the hand held beside the face, and oral speech given at the same time. Some residential schools favored this method as offering two approaches to English—lipreading and finger-spelling—at the same time, with the hope that each would reinforce the other. Some schools also used signs and speech simultaneously in classroom teaching, so that the pupils might follow whichever method they found the easier, and so gain knowledge more rapidly. (Finger-spelling is always used in conjunction with signs, to express words for which there are no general signs.) (115)

On the other hand, most of the day schools and many of the residential tended more and more toward oral teaching alone. Many schools advocated a complete separation of the oral and manual departments, arguing that it was like "teaching them to swim in ankle-deep water" to expect pupils to develop speech unless they were surrounded by a speech atmosphere. (115, p. 42) In many schools manual language was banned entirely.

Emphasis was centered increasingly on the importance of earlier teaching, and nursery classes were attached to both residential and day schools for deaf children. As this early work proved its value, the age level for admission was gradually lowered until, in some Centers, children are accepted as early as one year of age.

With this development came a turn towards a more natural synthetic approach to teaching speech. The Lexington School in New York was a leading proponent of natural speech and language presented in wholes rather than in parts. (200)

All avenues of multi-sensory approach were used, in every way the ingenuity of the teachers could contrive. There were various symbols and phonetic arrangements of letters, such as the Northampton Chart, to help a deaf child visualize the sounds of a printed word he had never heard. There were color codes to indicate the manner in which he should produce these sounds. There were diagrams and systems of marking to visualize for him the structure of a sentence and the organization of language, such as the Barry Five Slate System, The Fitzgerald Key, and the Wing Symbols. (115; 148)

At the upper end of the scale, we must place Gallaudet College, founded as a small private school in 1856 by Amos Kendall, who recruited for its head Edward Miner Gallaudet, the son of the famous Thomas Hopkins Gallaudet. It became, under his leadership, the only college exclusively for deaf students. In the classrooms of Gallaudet College, oral speech, finger-spelling and signs are used all at the same time, in the hope that the students may acquire knowledge by whichever means they can grasp most readily.

Situated in Washington, D.C., and supported by the Federal Government, this college offers unique opportunities in higher education for young deaf people.

At about the turn of the century, a new emphasis entered into the education of the deaf that was to have far-reaching effects. Systematic study of deaf children revealed that very few were totally deaf. Max A. Goldstein, a noted otologist, in the United States, was a strong advocate of the importance of residual hearing. He also developed and emphasized methods of making deaf children aware of sounds as vibration through the use of touch. He was much impressed by his contact with the work of Victor Urbantschitsch in Vienna, along these lines.

Working with St. Joseph's School for the Deaf, in St. Louis, Missouri, in 1897, he set up a series of acoustic exercises, giving each child fifteen minutes practice daily in sound stimulation. The results were most encouraging, in better speech and better comprehension of speech. (59,a, p. 15)

In 1914, Goldstein established The Central Institute for the Deaf in St. Louis, Missouri. This school was to be a private, orally-taught school for both residential and day pupils. Close cooperation was planned between teachers and scientists in otolaryngology, neurology, phoetics and acoustics. These plans have been carried out with constantly-increasing expansion. The research laboratories of Central Institute are adding vitally to our funds of knowledge in all these areas.

A nursery school was added in 1917 and a teacher training program in 1931. (59,b, pp. 38-41) There is also a full-scale department for children with language disorders of the aphasic type.

Goldstein pursued his "Acoustic Method" by every means he could devise. He used piano, accordion, organ, harmonica, and similar musical instruments, being especially interested in those that gave opportunity for combined tactile and auditory impressions. His "Simplex Hearing Tube" was in wide use in schools for deaf children. It consisted of a rubber tube, with a funnel at one end to catch the speaker's voice and a divided Y tube at the other, with metal tips to insert into the child's ears. For some time, Goldstein preferred this simple instrument to electric amplifiers because he felt the latter distorted the voice unnaturally. He finally admitted that for children with a severe loss it was necessary to have more amplification than the simple tube could provide and it would be better to sacrifice some naturalness for the sake of more volume.

Group hearing aids were introduced into classrooms, whereby the teacher had one mouthpiece and each child had an attached receiving unit. These were constructed both as a multiple Simplex tube, and with electric amplifiers. The electric amplification soon developed as the more satisfactory method and supplanted the simpler device. (59,b, p. 324) In recent years, Clarke School at Northampton, Massachusetts, has done exceptional work in auditory training with severely deaf children, with the use of powerful group hearing aids. (154)

In 1926, the acoustic engineers of the Bell Telephone laboratories, cooperating with committees of otologists, developed the audiometer for testing hearing. One type of audiometer used recordings of speech at controlled volume, with multiple earphones, so that a whole classroom of children could take the tests at the same time by writing their responses to what they heard. Foundation funds were obtained for sweeping surveys in the public schools. In this way, many childen with unsuspected moderate hearing losses were discovered and brought to the attention of medical and educational authorities.

Another type of audiometer was constructed to employ pure tones at measured pitches and controlled volume. By this means, a refined analysis could be made of the quality and quantity of each individual hearing loss and recommendations for remedies tailored to the individual need. (59,b, pp. 261-264)

In Great Britain, the trend of education for deaf children has been similar to that in the United States, with the educators and medical specialists cooperating closely in research studies and exchange of ideas.

The Education Act of 1893 placed the financial responsibility of the British schools for the deaf in the hands of the Department of Education, and made attendance compulsory from the age of seven. Some of the aspect of charity institutions was retained in the boarding schools until 1907, when this was abolished and the total responsibility accepted by the government.

As early as 1893, Dr. James Kerr Love, an aural surgeon of Glasgow, Scotland, demonstrated that fewer than ten percent of the children in the Glasgow Institution were totally deaf.

Day schools for deaf children grew up all over the country, especially in the urban areas where the number of deaf children made such special schools practical. Schools were divided according to the needs of the children. In Glasgow, at the insistence of Love, the children who were partially deaf and those who had acquired speech before deafness were separated, for their education, from the severely deaf.

In 1900, the London School Board established a special residential school at Hackney for the multiply-handicapped and deaf. In 1908, William Nelson, the Headmaster at Manchester, moved the slow-learning deaf children to a separate school. He also opened the residential school for the first time to children under six years of age, in 1912, and planned to have only six pupils in each oral class.

The Mary Hare Grammar School admitted only children of superior ability and set up a special curriculum to meet their needs.

Group hearing aid equipment was in use in the classrooms of the Royal Residential Schools of Manchester from 1932. Within the past few years, Great Britain has produced a new form of group hearing aid that is a fantastic improvement over any previous ones. An induction coil of wire is thrown around a classroom, playing field, or any other area in which deaf children are working. The children wear hearing aids tuned to the coil, without attached wires. The teacher or coach speaks quietly into his microphone, the amplification is evident to no one but the children wearing the special aids, but they hear clearly, while moving freely about the area.

The first Infant School was opened at Manchester in Worrall House in 1912, with Miss Irene R. Goldsack, the first teacher in charge. She left this position in 1919 to take charge of the University Department for the Education of the Deaf at Manchester University. Later she married Dr. Alex W. G. Ewing, (now Sir Alex) who became its first professor when, in 1949, the University established a chair for the Education of the Deaf.

Many schools had made provision by 1938 for the teaching of deaf children from the age of two years. All schools were becoming more child-centered in their philosophy and consequently taught more by experience lessons and less by old stereotyped methods.

Where the schools left off, missions to deaf adults, scattered over the British Isles, stood ready to help with problems of employment and social adjustment.

In both Great Britain and the United States, organizations of parents of deaf children, often in combination with the children's teachers, gathered continuing impetus and contributed much to the work. (54,a; 195; 196; 198)

For parents, who have discovered early that they have a deaf child, the John Tracy Clinic in Los Angeles has a school for preschool deaf children and their parents. The Clinic offers also a correspondence course for such parents who are not within reach of a proper school for their child or who wish to supplement the work of their school with lessons at home. Many isolated families the world around have taken advantage of these correspondence lessons to start a deaf baby on his road to education.

In France, a good deal of recent emphasis has been placed on psychological studies of deaf children, with a view to determining what differences might exist between them and normally-hearing children concerning their ability to use logical thinking and develop ideas and concepts. There has also been a systematic effort at diagnosis, to distinguish among such handicaps as hearing loss, auditory aphasia, and mental retardation, and to place the child in the proper educational situation. Oralism is the preferred method of teaching in all the schools. (181, p. 76; 199 pp. 165, 273, 278)

Madame Marcelle Charpentier, reporting to the World Congress for Deaf in Zagreb, Yugoslavia, in 1955, stated that France had recently begun extensive work with preschool deaf children beginning at the age of three. These children were considered too young to be separated from their families, so day classes were established for them, taught, for the most part, by teachers recruited from the field of nursery school education and given special training for teaching deaf children. The results were so gratifying that Charpentier predicted ". . . we are convinced that normal education in a normal environment will soon by the only method for deaf children. This will condition their happiness in adult life." (199, pp. 217-220)

A "Parent's Handbook" was published in 1955, compiled by the combined efforts of educational and medical experts, to enable parents in areas not in reach of these schools to begin the education of their young deaf children at home. (199, p. 224)

Beyond the pre-school age, the schools for the deaf in France have all been residential schools. (181, p. 76)

The importance of early discovery of hearing loss led to the establishment of Children's Audiology Centres, notably the one attached to the Paris National Institute for Deaf-Mutes, and the Regional Institute of Phono-Audiology of the University of Bordeaux. (199, pp. 10, 111) Hearing aids are in common use, both as individual, wearable aids and as group amplifiers in the classrooms. (199, p. 218)

In Germany, in 1920, the Malisch-Ratibor method of teaching speech by whole word and phrase units began to take the place of the older Vatter method of approach by articulation of single sound elements. (150, p. 268)

With the Nazi regime in 1933, the education of the handicapped took a different place in the scheme of things. Books on special education were ordered burned, and many of them were. Educators, some of them, reversed their thinking to fit into the new order.

Paul Schumann, who in 1927 had participated in a celebration in Leipzig honoring Heinicke, the father of education of the deaf in Germany, and had collaborated in a collection of his works, (114,a;b) now published an article in a professional magazine, in which he set matters in line with the new policy.

His subject was the place of the deaf in the New Reich and the question he asked was whether schools for the deaf were justified for the welfare of the State. It was his opinion that the education of the deaf was not without results, but that because of his language problem, it was more difficult for a deaf person to submerge his interests and lose himself in the whole state, no matter how intelligent or well-educated he might be. The quality of his work might not be affected, but his usefulness as a member of the national-socialistic state was curtailed. "Above all, he cannot serve in the army, and most of the women cannot bear children, being prevented from propagating their defect by the sterilization law. The deaf, therefore, never can be full citizens, but merely German subjects." (173, p. 201)

He also asked, "What is the value of the education of the deaf in the general scheme of education?" His answer was that "we may have clarified a few questions," but nobody could say that psychology, medicine, or pedagogy would have suffered much without it. So the only justification was social, that the deaf might take their place in the community, and to this extent society was responsible. But, he stated, there were limits to this responsibility, and it was a "biological sin" not to observe these limits, as was the case with the "Christian sentimentality" in favor of schools for the handicapped at the expense of public schools for normal children. It was his contention that the parents of "biologically inferior" children should pay the full price for their education, rather than penalize the parents of healthy children, who should be educated at State expense.

It was also the duty of the schools, he felt, to educate the deaf to a complete acceptance of the policies of the New State and to a submergence of their individualities in the totality of the new nation. The school for the deaf, therefore, in the New Germany would occupy an entirely different place.

The article closed with a ringing call to the German teacher of the deaf for his unconditional cooperation and his support of Hitler in the completion of "his tremendous task." (173)

After World War II, the German schools for deaf children took up where they had left off and began, as rapidly as they were able, to follow the same trends of progress taken in other nations. They emphasized early preschool training and maximum use of residual hearing. This is true in both the Eastern and Western Zones of Germany. (15, p. 270; 199, p. 225) Although still housed in corners of bomb-damaged buildings, the youngsters they teach are alert and eager, speaking good, intelligible German.

The schools in The Netherlands were taking the same direction. Reports by Dr. Henk C. Huizing, at the Audiological Center of the University of Groningen and Dr. A. Van Uden from the Institute of St. Michielsgestel, indicate that the Dutch also have been emphasizing early training and day schools, with families of deaf children encouraged to move into the vicinity of the schools, so that the children need not be separated from their families. Hearing aids are in constant use. There naturally follows an approach to the teaching of speech and language that more and more parallels that of hearing children.

Current literature from other countries tells the same story. The Scandinavian countries have kept in close touch with their neighbors, and have often led the way in scientific discoveries and in developing improved methods of teaching. From Eastern Europe and Southern Europe come similar reports. In Russia, in South America, in India, China and Japan, the same influences are at work. (171; 180; 182; 183; 199)

International conferences of various educational, medical and scientific organizations are held frequently in various countries. To these come representatives from every country in the world, bringing reports of their own work and taking home what they have heard from their colleagues in other nations. It is not surprising, then, with this constant interchange, that the reports of the education of the deaf everywhere are beginning to take on a more uniform color.

But the most revolutionary change of all has come with the development of individual wearable hearing aids.

From early years, as individuals developed hearing loss from various causes, they struggled to retain their ability to understand speech for as long as they were able. All manner of ingenious mechanical devices were constructed in some design that would gather sound waves with greater efficiency and channel them into the ear with some degree of amplification. A simple variety of such an ear trumpet, which was popular in England in the early nineteenth century, was a polished ram's horn, silver-mouthed and ivory-tipped, which the listener held with the small ivory tip in his ear, while he extended the large end toward the speaker's mouth. (59,a,b)

Similar sound-collecting apparatus, such as a large, horn-shaped opening ending in a small, flexible tube, was sometimes built into the high back of an armchair, or into a box to place on a desk, for social or business discourse. But the portable devices were far more popular and often took fantastic shapes. One was an actual conch shell of large size, with the conical tip cut off and a vulcanite tube cemented to the opening. Others imitated the shape of the cochlea of the ear. Many had convolutions and bulges of various sorts to provide resonance chambers and increase amplification. There was a large, folding fan, for a vibrant surface, which a lady could hold to her ear, or use in the usual manner.

There were even binaural devices to aid hearing. Some were shaped like snails, shells, or small trumpets, and worn above the ears, attached by a thin, tempered spring across the head, the whole apparatus more-or-less concealed by the hair or a hat. One was a rather narrow, elongated trumpet, hidden under a man's beard, with tubes to both ears to carry the sound.

For more elegant wear, the men had a pair of sound receptors in a tall silk hat, and the ladies had theirs in a magnificent tortoise-shell comb. In each case there were flexible tubes to both ears.

For bone conduction, there were various sound conductors to be held in the teeth. A flexible sheet of vulcanite was fitted with a handle and cords to control the degree of convexity of the surface, while the edge was pressed against the upper teeth. This was called an Audiphone, and was invented by R. S. Rhodes of Chicago in 1879. (59,b, p.347) The Japanese made an Otacoustic Fan, in about 1880, that was constructed of lacquered sheets of silk or vegetable fiber, with a flange of German silver added to the dental contact edge. Another modification was The Osteophone by C. M. Thomas of Philadelphia, Pa. This was a large receiving diaphragm, to be held at the body and away from the face so as to be less conspicuous. It was attached to a rod, bent in the form of a curved pipe-stem and held firmly in the teeth.

Paladino's sound conductor was a metal rod, eighteen to twenty-four inches long, with a metal disc on one end to be held in the listener's teeth, and a thin, circular metal arc on the other end, which was placed on the larynx of the speaker. (59,b, p. 346)

In 1900, Dr. Ferdinand Alt, an assistant in the Politzer Clinic of Vienna, produced the first electrical amplifying device for the use of hard-of-hearing people. It consisted of a small loudspeaker microphone, a telephone receiver and dry cell batteries, all con-

nected with wires. (59, a, p. 165) This was a major break-through
that lead to undreamed-of results.

Since this first electrical device of Alt, progress has been steadily
toward smaller, lighter instruments that could be worn at all times
with comfort and convenience. Earlier hearing aids were machines
that only a sturdy adult could manage. A unit containing the
microphone and amplifying tubes was worn in a vest pocket or in a
special harness on the chest. From this unit, wires went in two
directions, one to the receiver button in the ear, the other to a
heavy pack of batteries swung at the hip.

In the early 1940's, there began to appear on the market "one-
pack" hearing aids, small enough to contain batteries, amplifying
unit and microphone all in one case. This was a great convenience.
Hearing aids could now be worn even by children, so that they
need not leave the function of their ears behind them when they
leave the multiple amplifiers on their schoolroom desks. Still, for
very young children with severe hearing losses, the more powerful
aids were frequently so heavy that the weight of them noticeably
pulled down growing little shoulders.

With the development of the transistor to replace the vacuum
tube, hearing aids have become astonishingly small and light,
without sacrifice of power and quality. They can now be worn with
ease and comfort by anyone, including babies. Clarity and fidelity
of reproduction of sound have also improved. Every way is being
sought to restore sound and speech to as close a facsimile of normal
hearing as can be done.

A most dramatic development recently is the growing use of hearing aids binaurally. Two hearing aids are placed one on each side of
the head, behind the ears, so that sound is picked up from the normal position of the two ears on the head, and received by both ears
simultaneously, in the natural way. In addition, the constant static
distortion, clothing noises and muffling created by wearing the instrument in a pocket are eliminated.

The results in ability to interpret and comprehend sound and
speech, and the resulting improvement in the use of speech is most
dramatic and encouraging. This is especially true in young children
who, lacking hearing, have lacked, therefore, the capacity for
developing normal imitative speech. The long tortuous process of
building word on word, sometimes even sound on sound is
hastened and eased for them and their teachers almost beyond
belief.

These hearing aids are becoming so efficient that some powerful
enough to overcome severe hearing losses can be worn happily by

a baby at ten months of age. The predictions are that, as techniques improve, they will be fitted at younger and younger ages.

The hearing aids are fastened, one on each end of a light steel band encased in a nylon sleeve, which fits snugly on a child's head. A little girl may wear them pinned in her hair with barettes. Adults sometimes simply hang theirs over their ears on plastic hooks, or wear them built into the bows of their glasses.

The same improvements permit fitting a bone conduction aid on a baby with congenital atresia. With a bone conduction receiver at one end of the band and a powerful little hearing aid at the other, connected by a cord threaded through the nylon sleeve, such a child can hear and grow normally from babyhood in speech and language development while he waits out the years of growth necessary for him, until the surgeons can open the closed ear canals and let sound into the waiting ears.

So the road ahead for the education of the deaf becomes constantly brighter. Improved scientific techniques as well as increased professional and public awareness bring hearing loss to the attention of doctors and educators at constantly earlier ages. Improved modern hearing aids bring these little children up out of silence to a closer and closer approach to adequate hearing, while their language and speech training is begun at such an early age that the inevitable time lag with its problems of frustration and regression can now be almost eliminated. This makes possible the use of more normal techniques and materials in teaching deaf children, and consequently their increasing assimilation in the education of normally-hearing children.

The child today who is born with a hearing loss can look forward to a warm, happy acceptance in his family and his community, to a rich and complete education, and to full citizenship in society.

Chapter 10

UPDATE
1960-1980 in the U.S.

S. Richard Silverman

We can say with confidence that the period 1960-1980 witnessed a more intensive and broader assault on the "barriers of silence" than any other comparable period in history. The primary forces contributing to the assault were the dynamic social ambience of the era, the accelerating deinsularization of the field and a deepening consciousness of its professional status and identity. Although these forces were by no means unrelated, it is convenient to delineate them for purposes of exposition.

THE SOCIAL CLIMATE 1960-80

Mounting dissatisfaction with their place in the national scheme of things on the part of various identifiable minorities, notably blacks, surfaced conspicuously. The emergence of vigorous, militant, persistent demands for rights—civil, social, economic—was a reality that has left few, if any, facets of our national life untouched including, as we shall see, activities related to deafness and the deaf. Dissatisfaction and its epiphenomenon "advocacy" were expressed in a variety of dramatic ways, however much we may be disposed to judge them and their consequences. Violence, demonstrations, appeal to the courts and ultimately to the constitution were responses to limited or non-access to the political process, to "quality" education, to rewarding employment, and to suitable housing. This was viewed as an aberration of the "American dream."

The author acknowledges with appreciation the cooperation in the preparation of this chapter of Dr. E. Ross Stuckless, director, Office for Integrative Research, National Technical Institute for the Deaf, Rochester Institute of Technology.

168

There appeared to be a pervasive distrust, especially by young people, of existing institutions—political, social, business, educational and even of marriage and the family. Whatever its roots, an unpopular war in far away Vietnam, a failure of social action to achieve trumpeted expectations, political corruption, preoccupation with self ("my thing"), its reality was not to be doubted. A frequent expression of distrust was a demand for "accountability" of existing institutions and in some instances for scrapping them. For example, there is a continuing clamor for dismantling of residential and specialized, or as some would term them "segregated," facilities for the handicapped. It seemed that the "establishment" needed to be goaded to action if not rudely shaken up. Residential schools for the deaf were not entirely immune to this clamor.

Sensing the mood of the times, deaf people, parents of deaf children, active professionals and other interested individuals and groups were moved to expressions of their dissatisfactions, more often than previously, in forums beyond their own conventional contexts. Concern was voiced about poor academic achievement of graduates of schools for the deaf, limited career opportunities for deaf adults and non-participation by deaf persons in the affairs of their communities. Pronouncements as to the causes of this morbid state of affairs varied with those making them. Frequently cited were delayed identification of hearing impairment, ineffective prevailing modes of communication in schools, inadequately prepared teachers and other professionals, neglect of residual hearing, inordinate pupil-teacher ratios, unsatisfactory organization and administrative arrangements, employer discrimination of handicapped persons, lack of applied research, and public ignorance and indifference to deaf people reflected in meager community support. Such a wide spectrum of rhetoric suggested implicitly that the cause was not unitary or that the stated causes were of unequal or even questionable validity (Babbibge, 1965; "Colorado Conference," 1967).

Slogans like "The New Frontier" and "The Great Society" marked the political and social rhetoric of the 60's. During this period, a multitude of federally sponsored national conferences and other forums dealt with various aspects of deafness. Some brought representatives of different disciplines together to effect better coordination of services to the hearing-impaired child and adult, e.g., education and rehabilitation, education and audiology. Some were "state of the art" meetings, e.g. the "Colorado Conference" (1967) which addressed broad issues in education of the deaf, the "New Orleans Conference" (1965), which brought together social scientists representing numerous disciplines, all active in research on deafness. Others focused on particular issues and needs, e.g., teacher preparation, interpreting, vocational education, adult rehabilitation services. Still others were national workshops for service providers such as religious workers, social workers, psychologists, and, of course, teachers. These are just a few.

Several of these national meetings laid the base for enactment of new legislation. Some led to more effective implementation of existing laws and regulations. Others led to upgraded professional standards and certification requirements. These meetings crystalized issues and, in a sense, were a vehicle of advocacy for improving educational and rehabilitation services to the hearing impaired. They were also catalysts for the emergence of several new national organizations. The Registry of Interpreters for the Deaf (RID), founded in 1965, by 1980 numbered around 5,000 members, and had certified about 2,500 persons as interpreters. The American Deafness and Rehabilitation Association (ADARA) has its roots in one of these meetings and within 15 years had a membership approaching 1,000.

Two major parent organizations took on national significance during this period. The International Parents Organization (IPO) was formed as an affiliate of the Alexander Graham Bell Association for the Deaf, and the International Association of Parents of the Deaf (IAPD) was founded and affiliated with the National Association of the Deaf (NAD).

The time was ripe for unprecedented federal legislation which ushered in what was fundamentally a period of rising expectations and entitlements amply sustained by legislative sanction and fiscal support. Among the more significant legislative actions and their intent were the following:

85-905 (1958) - Captioned films for the deaf.

87-276 (1961) - Support to higher institutions of education for programs of preparing teachers of the deaf - enhancement of professional stature through involvement in peer review.

88-164 (1963) - Absorbed teacher training provisions of 87-276 and added provisions for advanced training at the doctoral level. Legislation authorizing the Vocational Rehabilitation Administration to support advanced training in research and administration was enacted at this time including what was termed Leadership Training.

89-36 (1965) - Established the National Technical Institute for the Deaf as integral unit of the Rochester Institute of Technology, enabling deaf students to take advantage of the influence of an outstanding technical institution of higher learning - a significant model for post-secondary education of the deaf. As of 1980, there were almost 1,000 students enrolled and many deaf graduates had already found employment in fields previously unavailable to them.

89-10 (1966) - Handicapped Child Benefit and Education Act - provided grants to the states for education of children in elementary and secondary schools, grants for the purchase of instructional materials, support of innovative programs, and policies to strengthen departments in the special education area - included a statutory National Advisory Committee on the Handicapped. There also was a statutory National Advisory Committee on Education of the Deaf established to advise on national policy specifically dealing with education of the deaf.

89-313 (1966) - Provided for direct support earmarked for the handicapped to the states.

89-694 (1966) - Provided for establishment of Model Secondary School for the Deaf on the campus of Gallaudet College to serve students from the District of Columbia and nearby regions and to provide "models" for improving secondary education for the deaf, and also 91-587 (1969) for the establishment of a model elementary school for the deaf (Kendall School) at Gallaudet College.

90-538 (1969) - Handicapped Children's Early Education Assistance Act - provided project grant funds for experimental preschool and early education programs for handicapped children.

91-61 (1969) - Provided for establishment of a National Center on Educational Media and Materials for the Handicapped and to facilitate the use of new educational technology in programs for handicapped persons.

91-230 (1969) - Provided for centers for serving deaf-blind children.

Section 504 of 93-112 (1973) - This amendment to the Rehabilitation Act led to regulations pertaining to equal employment opportunities for handicapped persons and access to services available to the general public.

94-142 (1975) - Education for All Handicapped Children Act - often associated with "mainstreaming," required education of all handicapped children in a "least restricted environment," an "individualized educational program" (IEP) determined by school people and parents, "due process" in case of difference of opinion, and auxiliary supportive help where needed.

Although this brief list has concentrated on legislation focusing on education, it is important to point out that other agencies were authorized to deal with other needs or target populations. The Vocational Rehabilitation Administration and its successor agencies liberally supported research, demonstration, training and service programs for the adult deaf. The National Institute of Neurological Diseases and Blindness, later to become the National Institute of Neurological and Communicative Disorders and Stroke, has supported training of promising young investigators and research in basic and clinical sciences which promises to increase our understanding of the biomedical and psychoacoustic aspects of

deafness on which advances in diagnosis and treatment undoubtedly depend (Eagles, 1975).

The foregoing is not intended to be an exhaustive list, nor does it
touch on legislation enacted at state and local levels, but documents
the tangible impact on deaf persons of the social climate of the
period 1960-80.

AN ISLAND NO MORE

The persistent insularity that characterized the education of the
deaf (or hearing impaired, if you will) since its beginning, when it
was in the hands of a dedicated but professionally inbred few, is no
more. The developments cited in the previous section contributed
greatly to concern for the deaf by a growing aggregation of interested groups and individuals. Among these were audiologists,
educators, engineers, government at all levels, linguists, parents,
philanthropists, phoneticians, physicians, psychiatrists,
psychologists, rehabilitation counselors, scientists, writers and,
very importantly, deaf persons themselves.

We turn now to a briefly annotated, but by no means
exhaustive, catalogue of the more important trends that comprise
the more general deisolating trend. These trends reflect directly or
indirectly the influence of the kinds of persons mentioned above
and here and there suggest that we are in the midst of a transition
from intuitive approaches (many of them ingenious) and largely
based on experience, to instructional, clinical and rehabilitative
procedures derived from scientific investigations. Nevertheless, we
need to recognize that there are still great open spaces between
scientifically determined facts that have been demonstrated to be
applicable to instruction and rehabilitation. Approaches based
primarily on experience still properly occupy an indispensable
place in professional efforts. However, it is to be hoped that the
trend to deinsularization will contribute productively to mutually
stimulating communication between investigators and practitioners
and even to their active collaboration in attacking the remaining
barriers of silence. The promise of this consequence is more or less
implicit in the trends herein delineated.

Prevention of Deafness: As important as any concern in achiev-
ing the conquest of deafness is its prevention. Most characteristics
of the hearing-impaired persons who have been the primary
historical focus of this book have been impairments related to their

inner ears. The key concept is that sensory cells are not replaced in kind. Absent sensory cells may have never been present as in the case of genetic failure in development or in intrauterine or other infections or they may have been present and then lost. Hereditary deafness is now understood as a genetic problem and its associated syndromes and linkages have been rather well established but prevention, as of now, is not possible (Fraser, 1976; Konigsmark & Gorlin, 1976). Genetic counseling may be helpful and expanding knowledge may enlighten us to the level of confidence with which we can now diagnose and counsel about genetic matters. Of course, effective counseling recognizes the requirement of mature sensitivity to the ethical, moral and psychological factors involved in the delicate process of family planning.

On the other hand, prevention of deafness by immunization is possible to an increasing degree through prevention or limitation of the various infectious diseases that may impair hearing such as the familiar diseases of childhood. Among these are scarlet fever, mumps and measles. Prevention is also accomplished through successful treatment of certain diseases that are a threat to hearing, prominent among which are bacterial meningitis and neonatal kernicterus (jaundice of the newborn). Identification and avoidance of ototoxic drugs has been helpful too.

A viral disease that has had a grave and lasting impact on the education of many deaf children and their overall management is rubella. If a pregnant woman contracts this disease, particularly in the first trimester of pregnancy, the virus may enter the fetus and cause very serious damage not only to the developing ear but to eyes, heart, central nervous system, or any combination of these. Although these effects of maternal rubella were first observed in Australia during the period 1941-45, the unnerving jolt to the field was the epidemic of 1964-65 (Calvert 1969). Of the children born in those years who were subsequently enrolled for special education 41% in 1964 and 34% in 1965 were reported as having rubella caused deafness, many with additional handicaps (Trybus, Karchmer, Kerstetter and Hicks, 1980). Awareness that the so-called "rubella bulge" would in the 80's require expanded provision for postsecondary education and rehabilitation, and unfortunately for some, continuing custodial care, led to the organization of a national working conference on the subject in September, 1980 attended by a variety of qualified professionals and deaf and deaf-blind persons. An issue of the *American Annals of the Deaf* (Stuckless, 1980) is devoted entirely to the Conference presentations. On the encouraging side, efforts to develop an immune serum were successful and it was licensed for general distribution in 1969. And as a result the predicted epidemic for 1972 did not occur.

Early Identification of Deafness: If deafness cannot be prevented or succcessfully treated, appropriate constructive measures need to be instituted based on an understanding of its consequences for the affected individual. Basic is the recognition of the potential benefits of shaped sensory experience for a plastic, maturing nervous system. The benefits are more likely to be realized if deafness is identified as early in a child's life as possible. It is interesting to note that Dalgarno, whose work is discussed in Chapter 5, suggested as long ago as 1680 that "There might be successful addresses made to a dumb child, even in his cradle" (Dalgarno, 1680). But unfortunately deafness has generally not been identified and diagnosed until the infant is 20 months or older, usually coincidental with the recognition that the child's language is delayed (Bergstrom, 1976, Davis, 1965; Elliott and Armbruster, 1967; Mencher, 1976).

A number of general approaches dominate procedures aimed at identification of deafness in neonates and infants. One is based on the presentation of a specifiable stimulus, usually a high frequency pure tone, followed by observer judgment as to whether a response has occurred. Among the criticisms of this approach are low-cost benefits for expended effort, false positives, varying infant states not accounted for by episodic testing, questionable competence of observers and the possibility of inducing anxiety in families based on meager evidence. A method that promises to overcome some of these criticisms, especially as it eliminates the need for a human observer, is the Crib-o-gram (Simmons, 1976). The basic elements of the completely automated system begin with a motion-detecting transducer on each crib. The output from these transducers is fed to a multi-channel strip chart recorder. Test sounds are introduced and are scored by comparing the motor activity of the baby during the baseline pre-sound recording against activity changes immediately after the test sound.

Another approach to early identification of hearing impairment is the identification of "at risk" infants as determined by history and physical examination. Among the recommended screening criteria are a history of genetically determined childhood hearing impairment, rubella or other non-bacterial intrauterine fetal infection, defects of ear, nose and throat, low birthweight and any chemical concentration that is potentially toxic. Whatever turns out to be the method or methods of choice, it is fortunate that the search *per se* has underlined the need for and the value of early identification. This, along with public education of all concerned with infants should improve our screening score (Feinmesser and Tell, 1976; Simmons, 1978).

Not only is progress being made in identification of deafness but, as we follow a screened-out child, increasingly refined assessment of the nature and degree of hearing loss is within reach - the middle ear by impedance testing, the inner ear by electrocochleography and the neural transmission and central nervous system by evoked response methods (Bradford, 1975). More attention, too, is being paid by audiologists to those items of assessment that may be pertinent to remedial and educational management such as perception of patterns, ability to use minimal acoustic cues, attentiveness to sound and differential sensitivity to signal frequency, intensity and duration.

The need to be alert to handicaps additional to hearing impairment is emphasized by findings of the Office of Demographic Studies at Gallaudet College in the U.S.A. Approximately 30% of hearing-impaired children in special classes have one or more additional handicaps. Ranking high among these handicaps are brain damage, low vision, mental retardation and emotional-behavioral problems (Gentile and McCarthy, 1973).

Early Education, the Communication Controversy: Early identification and subsequent continuing assessment are preludes to early education. The idea that early education (by parents and teachers) is essential if we are to improve our performance, is just about universally accepted. Students of linguistics and the psychology of learning have stressed the importance for language acquisition of the time from birth through the first four or five years. This lends support to everyday observations. Empirical-descriptive studies suggest stages at which hearing children induce the phonologic, syntactic and semantic rules of language. Of interest is the hypothesis that human beings inherit, rather than learn, some abilities for perceiving speech sounds. Human infants who have not yet begun to speak are able to perceive speech sounds and subsequently lose the ability to hear contrasts between speech sounds that are not differentiated in the language they eventually speak. This suggests an attrition of potential communication skills if there is no environmental stimulation of genetically determined capability. How much this capability can be modified is probably determined by the kind and amount of environmental stimulation and the time of life or "critical period" during which it is provided.

Common to all methods or general strategies of early "management" or education, is the premise that the early years are optimal for establishing the foundation for the child's acquisition of communication and his emotional or "affective" maturation. And what happens then is more than likely to determine the course of his subsequent formal education, particularly its setting, its relative emphasis on certain modes of communication, the preparation of its teachers, and its explicit goals.

A list of what may loosely be called methods is obviously beyond the scope of this chapter but it is important for an understanding of the current scene to present some general features of two differing methods that curiously enough rest on the same basic premise. One of these exploits the fact that the primary, although not always exclusive, channel for speech and language development is auditory and that the input is fluent, connected speech. The terms "Auditory-Oral," "Acoupedic," "Natural" and "Unisensory" are conventional synonyms for the same fundamental method or they designate variations within the same general framework (Beebe, 1953; Griffiths, 1974; Ling, 1964; Pollack, 1970; Simmons-Martin, 1972).

The method stresses *maximum* use of the auditory channel, however much its sensitivity is reduced. The more enthusiastic among its followers say "There is no such thing as a totally deaf child", and "Every remnant of hearing is usable for developing oral communication" which incidentally is an explicit goal, the attainment of which is crucial for the most desirable development of the child. However, the restricted auditory sensitivity of the hearing-impaired child reduces the redundancy and the linguistic cues of the language available to him. Nevertheless, it is argued, there may still be sufficient auditory and visual cues to facilitate inductive acquisition of the rules of speech and language. If all requirements of the method are satisfied, practical oral speech and language competence should be acquired, thus paving the way for the child's integration or "mainstreaming" in schools for hearing children with all the advantages for subsequent economic and social self-realization. The impressive number of hearing-impaired persons who have achieved these goals is inspiring and should, so the reasoning goes, influence our aspirations accordingly.

Nevertheless, it is also argued that we need to anticipate realistically that this method will not be satisfactory for all children. Even if the major focus of a program for an individual child is oral competence and our goal is maximal exploitation of the opportunities of the world of the hearing, alternate methods or modifications need to be considered, for example, those that stress multisensory stimulation, deliberate development of and drill on speech sounds and their combinations, smaller units of speech input and more structured language instruction. The point is that we need to know if, when and how to intervene to change a general strategy that may have seemed promising at the outset.

Another "method" that proceeds from the premise of the importance of early education is probably best subsumed under the rubric "Total Communications" (Garretson, 1976). The primary feature of this approach is that all modes of communication are recommended from the beginning. It advocates the inclusion of manual forms of communications. Proponents stress that sole reliance on residual hearing and speechreading for communication results in ambiguous, deficient, or no communication at all, which, in turn, retards cognitive development. Furthermore, poor communication between parent and child may lay the groundwork for psychological difficulties. Continuing experience, it is maintained, confirms the reality and the necessity of an active "deaf community" which can attract deaf adults who find security in its sanctions, its modes of communication, its opportunities for social expression and its organized advocacy of causes beneficial to deaf persons. Therefore, this is to be preferred to a goal of "integration" into "hearing society." And it is most likely to be attained by the Total Communication approach instituted as early as possible. As of now there appears to be no universal agreement on what constitutes applied Total Communication.

Nevertheless, although some school systems provide a choice of communication modes for instructional purposes, the trend appears to be toward Total Communication. The controversy over modes of communication not only among aural, oral and manual forms, or combinations of them, but also over variations within a particular basic mode is by no means settled. It is encouraging, however, that numerous investigations are under way to study not only the linguistic, conceptual and economic effects of modes of communication for deaf persons but also their influence on such features of personality as emotional maturity and self and group identity. A brief review of current trends in key modes of communication follows.

COMMUNICATION

Speech: The paramount factors influencing instruction in speech during the period were the exploitation for speech development of the early years of the life of a hearing-impaired child, recognition of the potential use of the auditory system as the method of initial choice for speech training, and emphasis on imposition of structure on a developmental sequence rather than stress at the outset on remediation.

Although systematic auditory training has been enthusiastically championed by a few people it was not widely practiced in classrooms. It is interesting to speculate why. In this writer's opinion the more significant among them are skepticism about the cost effectiveness of concentrated auditory training especially for the severely and profoundly deaf, emphasis on evaluating training only on receptive skills to the exclusion of its contribution to speech acquisition and improvement, nonreinforcing aural-oral environments, indifference to thorough audiologic assessment of auditory capacity, and little early identification and consequent use of amplification. Other factors include the unavailability, at least in the earlier period, of convenient, durable, wearable and acoustically effective hearing aids, failure to stress or even include aural approaches in teacher training, paucity of materials of demonstrated value for structuing the training and integrating it with speech, language and academic instruction and just a persistent annoyance on the part of some experienced professionals with the "exaggerated claims" advanced by ebullient advocates of an acoustic approach. The weight of these factors or combinations of them undoubtedly varied with local attitudes and circumstances (Silverman, 1981).

Unlike the initial emphasis on articulation, the concept of developmental sequence rests on the recognition that phonation and prosody precede precise articulation. Children appear to learn intonation patterns before they learn segmental features (Weir, 1966). Thus, the general sequence requires the child first to vocalize, to control vocal duration and pitch and to produce vowels and consonants in that order (Calvert and Silverman, 1975; Ling, 1976).

Students of speech of deaf children have been greatly stimulated by the development of improved tools and methods for the investigation of speech as an acoustic event. We now have electronic techniques for analyzing and synthesizing speech, for making it available for visible and tactual display, and for manipulating it by selective filtering, frequency transposition, and temporal expansion and compression. These should aid our analysis of the perceptual features of speech and guide us in its appropriate tailoring for the benefit of the speech development of children whose range of perceptual cues of speech is severely limited.

Speechreading (Lip Reading): Investigators of speechreading have begun to demonstrate what teachers have observed for some time. Skill in speech reading may be a composite of perceptual efficiency including ability to perceive speech elements rapidly, visual acuity, attention span, peripheral vision and visual memory, all of this along with synthetic ability. The speechreader augments the words and phrases he can identify with whatever linguistic and situational cues are available to discern the gist of the message. In the case of children especially, linguistic proficiency is fundamental (Perry and Silverman, 1978).

Ingenious attempts have been made to relate intelligence, educational achievement, hearing level, time of onset of deafness, linguistic and perceptual skills, and personality to judged or measured speechreading ability. Although there are promising leads here and there, and the value of speechreading as a complementary element in bisensory communication is being demonstrated, there is still no clear pattern of relationships.

Hearing: The data on the hearing status of hearing-impaired students in special classes and schools in the U.S. reported by the Office of Demographic Studies at Gallaudet College point to a substantial number of children with hearing which, if cultivated, would facilitate their development of useful oral communication. The data indicate that 45% of hearing-impaired children in special classes are reported to have hearing levels of 84 decibels or less in the three speech frequencies. Fostering the use of residual hearing has been, first, the availability of improved hearing aids which can now be worn conveniently on the person, and second, our increasing knowledge of speech perception and its exploitation. Impressively efficient transducers, coupled to compact circuitry, produce a reasonably faithful amplified speech signal that is useful even for the child with a small residuum of hearing. Auditory experience, even of the prosodic features, sometimes referred to as the suprasegmental features of speech, if frequent enough, can help significantly in the reception, and consequently in the production of speech. Experiments have shown too that speechreading is enhanced by acoustic cues. We anticipate that hearing aid design and engineering will keep pace with our knowledge of speech perception. The aim is to transmit the crucial information-bearing features of the speech signal and to eliminate or reduce those that make little or no contribution. Attempts are underway, too, to implant an induction coil device (cochlear implants) in the ear to transmit an electrical signal to the auditory nerve of postlingually profoundly deaf patients. Surgical procedures have been successful and, as of now, the promise of these devices have their enthusiasts and their skeptics.

Manual Communication: The trend toward Total Communication, of which manual communication is a dominant feature, has stimulated a growing academic and professional interest in all forms of manual communication. An important trend is the continuing analysis of the structure of American Sign Language. That its codification in written form was possible grew out of the recognition by Stokoe and his collaborators that every sign could be analyzed into at least three components: (1) the **place** on the body where the sign is made; (2) the **shape** of the hands making the sign; (3) the **movement** of the hand or hands. In a sense, these components called **cheremes** may be analagous to phonemes of oral language. Lexical-semantic and syntactic linguistic features are also being investigated (Mayberry, 1978; Stokoe, Casterline and Croneberg, 1965). Worthy of note here is that investigators of signed languages have found that there are primary linguistic systems, passed down from one generation of deaf people to the next, which have developed into autonomous languages and are not derived from spoken languages. Thus the properties of visual-gestural channels of transmission are being studied. It is claimed that the study of language transmitted by another modality should enhance the understanding of the structure of language, its acquisition, related cognitive processes and contraints on linguistic form (Bellugi and Studdert-Kennedy, 1980).

Educators of the deaf agree that the acquisition and use of the English language are essential to the education of deaf children and to their interaction with the English speaking and writing community. Therefore, a variety of sign systems have been developed and introduced to children as manual-visual equivalents to oral language. Nevertheless, the proportional use of fingerspelling and signs, the choice of a language-gesture or concept-gesture relation and its effect on language learning, the probability that the prosodic features of speech so important for optimum use of residual hearing are blurred when speech and manual forms are presented simultaneously, are among the many open questions. Fundamental questions pertain to processing of sign language, its "grammar" and its relation to spoken language, attainment of fluency by "non-native" signers, especially parents and teachers, and by interpreters in specialized fields.

Language: It is appropriate to discuss language in this section since it is the "stuff" of communication. The discipline of psycholinguistics has resulted in an almost exponential growth in the study of language — its structure, its acquisition, how it is taught and how it is evaluated. In historical retrospect of the past 20 years or so we find that initially child-language studies were dominated by grammatical formalism. Investigators studied how children acquire and internalize grammatical forms such as questions, passives, and negatives. This led to attempts to write content-free grammars of emerging child language. These were essentially based on distribution of words within children's utterances and made no reference to what their reasons for speaking might be. Equivalence of form rather than differences in meaning was the center of attention.

Rigid formalism came to be questioned with the recognition that it is necessary to study the context in which an utterance is produced in order to understand the meaning the child is trying to express. For example "baby water" may mean "the baby wants water," "the baby is in the water," "the baby spilled the water," etc. This suggested that we need to be concerned with the "semantic rules" that relate words or sentences to things and events.

Even this conceptualization had some gaps. The notion has developed that a complete description of what children are doing when they speak includes not only the actual forms produced and their context but the social use of that speech. Is that utterance a request for information? A casual comment? Or what? Does it take account of the knowledge the hearer shares or does not share with the speaker? Thus the forms, the content of intended meaning, and the special uses of speech have emerged as a tripartite focus of most current child-language study.

These investigations of normal language development have begun to influence our thinking if not our management and instructional practices. Evidence of application and results are not at hand probably because of the recency of findings, the issues related to them, and the undetermined significance they may have for language acquisition and instruction of hearing-impaired or learning-disabled children.

Concurrent with these notions and perhaps stimulated by them is interest in subtle interweaving of language and thought. The argument is advanced that cognitive development both precedes and enables language development. The aim here is to extract the child's cognitive understanding underlying language performance and to specify the nonlinguistic tasks.

The possible implications for the education of hearing-impaired children from research in the development of language of hearing children command our serious and earnest attention. It is conceivable that this work may influence, among other things, our modes of communication, the timing, sequencing and structuring of language input, our concepts of "correctness" of language production at various levels in a child's development, and our assessment of language competence and achievement. We may thus be led to hierarchical development as a point of departure for dealing with language disorders rather than pervasive remediation (Blackwell, 1978; Elliott, 1976; Kretschmer and Kretschmer, 1978; Silvermand, 1980; Streng, 1972).

EDUCATIONAL TRENDS

Educators of the hearing impaired were quick to take advantage of the major educational trends of the period, including the "technology" of education. Educators recognized "programed instruction" when it arrived on the scene in the early 1960's, and its successor "computer-assisted instruction" which was introduced in the late 1960's and early 1970's.

They sensed the possibilities of instructional television and introduced it into the classroom. They were prepared when "behavioral objectives" and later "competency-based instruction" entered the vernacular and the substance of education (forerunners of the "Individualized Educational Plan" or IEP which was given legal status in 1975 as a result of Public Law 94-142).

They anticipated perhaps before the general field, the mandate for "Career Education" in the 60's, generously funded by federal dollars. This, coupled with the Vocational Education Amendments of 1968 which specified the allocation of support to the vocational education of handicapped students, had an influence on secondary and postsecondary education of the hearing impaired in the 1970's.

Although educators of the deaf were slow to take advantage of the Community College movement in the post World-War II period, they recognized its possibilities beginning in the late 1960's, and extending throughout the 1970's. Community College-based programs for the hearing impaired proliferated until at the close of the 1970's there were at least 30 such programs, and perhaps another 20 programs based in four-year undergraduate institutions (Rawlings, Trybus, and Biser, 1981).

Among these is the National Technical Institute for the Deaf which was established by law in 1965. As an integral part of the Rochester Institute of Technology, NTID's enrollment in less than 15 years had grown to approximately 1,000 hearing-impaired students. Four regional programs were established with federal support in the late 1960's at St. Paul TVI in Minnesota, Seattle Community College, in Washington, California State University at Northridge, California, and Delgado Community College in Louisiana. In the meantime, Gallaudet College's enrollment had also increased substantially.

The net effect was a more than quadrupling in enrollment of deaf students in postsecondary programs, up to around 4,000 in 1980, most of whom were enrolled in career-oriented majors. The proportion of hearing-impaired high school graduates taking advantage of postsecondary educational opportunities, nearing 50%, today begins to approach that of normally hearing students.

We referred earlier to Public Law 94-142, The Education for All Handicapped Children Act of 1975. The 1970's will probably be best remembered (or "worst" remembered by its critics) for the passage and implementation of this legislation, commonly known as the "Mainstreaming" law. It is too soon to assess its full implications and the degree and extent of its impact.

THE IMPACT OF TECHNOLOGY

The unabating advances of technology are having a considerable impact on the lives of deaf persons. In the educational context we have already referred to advances in tools of audiologic assessment, and in hearing aids. Communication engineers have developed sensory aids that are designed to extract and transmit features of speech that are likely to facilitate speech perception and hence speech production. Visual displays of pitch, temporal dynamics, and transmission of distinctive features of phonemes to the skin illustrate the range of possibilities that are being investigated. Sensory aids may serve as vehicles for self-instruction, particularly in their role as "error detectors." They may be imaginatively designed to appeal to children's interests and motivate practice (Levitt and

Nye, 1971). Many of these devices are in the experimental or laboratory stage and their contribution to communication in real life situations needs to be carefully evaluated.

Visual and audiovisual media are being increasingly employed to aid instruction of all kinds and at all levels. The design of instruments, the procedures for their use and the creation of materials adapted to them have enlisted the attention of an imposing variety of workers interested in "mediated" instruction (Stepp, 1980). The overhead projector to be found in every progressive classroom and lecture hall is a conspicuous example of the application to instruction of media technology. Even the design of teaching spaces has begun to attend to the acoustic and lighting features that insure optimum accommodation to media equipment.

Thanks to the cooperation of the federally supported National Captioning Institute, the Public Broadcasting System, and the commercial broadcasting industry, television is now more accessible to the hearing impaired. Under a "closed-caption" system, a decoding device is required to enable the viewer to "tune into" the captions; otherwise no captions are displayed to distract the hearing viewer. Within a year of their becoming available in 1979, over 20,000 closed-caption adapters had been purchased for home use by an estimated 50,000 hearing-impaired viewers, and over 20 hours a week of captioned television had become available (Jensema and Fitzgerald, 1981).

Alexander Graham Bell would be pleased to know that his epochal invention, the telephone, is now increasingly accessible to deaf persons. In the early 60's a deaf physicist, R.H. Weibrecht, working with an old teletypewriter (TTY) invented a coupler that would send signals from the TTY across telephone lines to another TTY with a like coupler that would decode the signals and print the written message.

By 1980, a variety of telecommunication devices for the deaf (TDD's) had become commercially available, some of which are quite compact and portable, and there were 40,000 or more TDD's in hearing-impaired individual's homes and places of business. Many public agencies including police departments, medical facilities, and government offices (including the Internal Revenue Service) had acquired TDD's, offering hearing-impaired citizens greater access to community resources.

The burgeoning technology of the past two decades has contributed to an improved lifestyle for deaf people, while at the same time raising new questions for our attention. Should TDD's be made "computer-compatible?" Is computer-assisted instruction cost effective? Should captions be presented verbatim on film and TV and how does this relate to reading rate and reading level of the "average" deaf viewer?

PSYCHOSOCIAL DEVELOPMENTS

The Deaf Community: Anthropologists and sociologists generally have not applied their disciplines to deafness to the extent that psychologists and linguists have. The broadening of interest in the field of deafness may attract them to important social questions relating to deaf children and adults in the future.

Today, when we contemplate psychosocial developments anthropologically and from an aggregate point of view, we inevitably encounter the concept and the reality of the "deaf community." It appears rather convincingly well defined as a distinctive subculture whose members are attracted to it by the security it offers through its sanctions, its modes of communication and its opportunities for social expression (Schein, 1968).

As suggested earlier in this chapter, the civic, political, economic and social assertiveness of the deaf community has in recent years been encouraged by the amount and variety of legislation responsive to its wishes and addressed to its needs. In the tradition of American cultural pluralism, it advocates retention and public knowledge of its identity and at the same time resists limitation of its access to the larger arena of national life. The National Association of the Deaf exemplifies this spirit, penetrating virtually every sector affecting the deaf community. The deaf community serves its members through a variety of groups organized around such interests as religion, sports, recreation, theatre, social services, etc., and through them projects its identity to the public. Evidence of the latter is the provision of oral and manual interpreters at an increasing number of public events, captioning of television programs, public presentations by the National Theatre of the Deaf, and growing opportunities in the world of work for interaction with hearing persons.

This is emphatically not to say that all deaf or hearing-impaired persons identify actively or even at all with the deaf community. Many have accommodated to and participate in the world at large without recourse to support or dependence on reinforcement from groups in which deafness is the primary cohesive force. Since they are not identifiable or conspicuously visible members of the deaf community, they are generally not available to conventional sociological surveys and their frequent impressive and diverse accomplishments seldom, if ever, are entered into the aggregate data about deafness and the deaf.

Psychological Assessment: The search for valid and reliable tests and measures of intelligence, personality skills and achievement of deaf persons continues. Historically recognized limitations of the variety of available tests still challenge the test framer and test user. These include, among others, the influence on test results of language content, mode of instructions to test takers, differentiation of perception from cognition, familiarity of the tester with deaf children or adults, choice of norms (deaf or hearing) and interpretation of results, particularly the weight to be attached to them for such important purposes as school placement or career guidance.

The increasing number and kinds of psychologists addressing these issues may hasten their ultimate clarification to the satisfaction of all concerned, especially deaf persons themselves. Concentrated academic and professional training programs to prepare specialists in the "psychology of deafness" are evolving and their experience may eventually enhance knowledge of this complex subject (Craig and Barkauloo, 1968; Elliot, 1974; Furth, 1966; Stark, 1974; "New Orleans Conference", 1965).

Mental Health: There is a widely perceived need for salutary measures aimed at the mental health of deaf persons. Custodial care in state hospitals for the mentally ill where adequate communication with deaf patients was simply ignored is gradually giving way to appropriate inpatient and outpatient services (Rainer, Altschuler, Kallman, and Deming, 1963). Among these are facilities at the Rockland, New York Psychiatric Center, St. Elizabeth Hospital in Washington, D.C., Langley-Porter Neuropsychiatric Institute in San Francisco, and the Psychosomatic and Psychiatric Institute of Michael Reese Hospital in Chicago.

This all too brief commentary on psychosocial matters suggests persuasively that deaf persons do not constitute a homogeneous mass. They differ among themselves, as is the case with any other group of people, and it is the better part of caution to avoid the simplistic and hasty stereotyping that misleads the public and wrongly influences perception of their needs, their capabilities and their aspirations.

THE PROFESSION MATURES

Coincident and closely intertwined with the impact of powerful societal trends and the stimulation by vigorous deisolating influences on the barriers of silence has been what can best be described as a deepening consciousness of professional stature. To enhance, dignify and validate that stature required of "the profession" not only to respond to the forces but to seize all opportunities to shape them.

In the late 50's and early 60's, as we have noted, the possibility, indeed the strong probability of enactment of legislation at the national level to benefit the handicapped in unprecedented ways loomed large on the social and political scene. This aroused special interest groups to press for legislation that would benefit their constituencies. Leaders and friends of the groups realized that legislative action was facilitated if its advocates spoke with "one voice." It appears to be a cardinal principle of the legislative process that disparate points of view tend to retard or impede desired outcomes. The profession dealing with the education and rehabilitation of deaf persons certainly did not lack for disparate and conflicting views on how its tasks should be accomplished. The pages of this book attest to that. Nevertheless, the temper of the times encouraged submersion of differences, at least in public and political discourse, for the sake of the larger common good. This led to the establishment early in this period of the Council on Education of the Deaf composed of representatives of the three historically major organizations whose primary, if not exclusive, concern was the education of deaf children, namely, Convention of American Instructors of the Deaf, Alexander Graham Bell Association for the Deaf, and the Conference of Executives of American Schools for the Deaf (since renamed the Conference of Educational Administrators Serving the Deaf).

The formation of the Council was not just a symbolic gymnastic. Designated members testified in its name before important congressional committees concerned with deafness and the deaf. The Council also acted as the official host for the International Congress on Education of the Deaf held in Washington, D.C., in June, 1963, attended by over 2,200 participants from 52 countries (Doctor, 1964). Evidence of growing recognition of the profession was the federal financial support of this enterprise without which it could not be carried out. Also, consistent with the principle of professional self-regulation, the Council has taken on the responsibility of setting standards for professional training programs, and has established a mechanism for their accreditation, an activity that it currently administers.

The elaboration of the definition of the profession, both in breadth and in depth, proceeded at a rapid pace. Stimulated by the increase in pertinent knowledge and the ease of its exchange nationally, specialties began to emerge and to be institutionalized. Among these specialists were psychologists, audiologists, supervisors, counselors of all sorts, parent educators, psychiatrists, social workers, vocational placement specialists, oral and manual interpreters. Others included teachers qualified at specified age levels and in subject matter, administrators, media experts, instructors in speech and sign language, coordinators in public school systems, house parents, athletic coaches, legal aides, sex educators, demographers, and clergy-men and women. And it was inevitable that the specialists would soon group themselves into formal organizations or informal "networks" which in turn gave rise to conferences, workshops, and literature addressed to their interests and purposes. Of course, the trend to increased institutionalization of professional specialities is not unique to the field of deafness. It is happening, for better or worse, in all professions.

Maturation of the profession was by no means limited to the United States. Professional growth was international. This is amply documented by the International Congresses held in Washington in 1963, Stockholm in 1970, Tokyo in 1975, and Hamburg in 1980, as well as other international conferences of various groups, and increasing international academic, professional and citizen exchange. An International Congress Committee on Education of the Deaf was organized at the Tokyo Congress to solicit and evaluate proposals for future congresses and to advise about their organization and programs. Limitation of space and abundance of material has confined this update to the American context, but there is no question that American developments have been importantly influenced by exchanges with colleagues from other lands.

A combination of professional initiative and public interest led to the organization by the National Advisory Committee on the Education of the Deaf (mentioned earlier in this chapter), of a National Conference on the Education of the Deaf at Colorado Springs in April, 1967 attended by a broad representation of professional workers including many from allied fields ("Colorado

Conference'', 1967). The Conference report issued by the United States Department of Health, Education and Welfare set an agenda for action that is still in various states of implementation. Leading up to the Conference was the report of an advisory committee commissioned in 1964 by the Department to a study of the problems of the education of the deaf and of the programs in the nation which are directed at meeting them. It is jarring to quote the first sentence in the summary and recommendations of the report:

> The American people have no reasons
> to be satisfied with their limited
> success in educating deaf children
> and for preparing them for full
> participation in our society
> (Babbidge, 1965).

Would the social ambience and the deinsularization and maturation of the field discussed in this chapter cause a commission reporting in 1985 to write in a more commendatory vein? For all concerned with penetrating the barriers of silence that is the question.

Bibliography

BOOKS

1. Agricolae, Rodolphi Phrisii. *De Inventione Dialectica*, Anno MDLVII (1557). No publisher given.
2. Akerly, Samuel. *Elementary Exercises for the Deaf and Dumb.* New York: E. Conrad, 1821.
3. Anderson, Duncan. *A Graduated Vocabulary and Dictionary for the Use of the Deaf and Dumb.* London: Griffin, Bobin, and Co., 1861.
4. Alberti, Salomonis. *Oratio de Surditate et Mutitate.* Noriberg: M. Ernesto Helten-Bachio Mergenthu, ae anno 1591.
5. Amman, John Conrad: [a]*A Dissertation on Speech.* Originally printed in Latin, by John Walters, Amsterdam, 1700. Translator not given. London: Low, Marston, Low and Searle, 1873.
   [b] Amman, Jo. Conradi. *Surdus Loquens sive Dissertatio de Loquela.* Lugdieni Batavorum: Apud So. Arn. Langerak, 1727.
6. Antonio, D. Nicolao, Hispolensi. *Bibliotheca Hispana nova sive Hispanorum Scriptorum qui ab anno MD ad MDCLXXXIV Floruere.* Matriti apud Joachim de Ibarra, Typographum, Requim 1788, Tomus Primus.
7. Artistotle, [a]*The Works of.* Translated into English under the editorship of J. A. Smith and W. D. Ross. Vol IV, Historia Animalum, by D'Arcy Wentworth Thompson. Oxford: Clarendon Press, 1910.
   [b] ΑΡΙΣΤΟΤΕΑΗΣ. Aristotle *Opera Omnia, Graece et Latine.* Editore, Ambrosio Firmin Didot. Parisiis: Instituti Franciae Typographe, 1854.
8. Arnold, Thomas. [a]*Aures Surdis, The Education of the Deaf and Dumb.* London: Elliott Stock, 1879.
   [b] *Education of the Deaf, A Manual for Teachers.* Revised and rewritten by A. Farrer, second edition. London: Published by the National College of Teachers of the Deaf. Printed and sold by Francis Carter, 1923.

9. Arrowsmith, John Paunceforth. *The Art of Instructing the Infant Deaf and Dumb.* London: Taylor and Heasey, 1819.

10. Arsenian, Seth, Editor, *Rudolf Pintner.* Springfield, Massachusetts: 1951.

11. Augustini, Sancti Aurelii, Hipponensis Episcopi *Traditio Catholica,* Saecula IV-V Opera Omnia, Tomus Decimus, contra Julianum, Horesis Pelagianea defensorum, Liber Tertius, Caput IV-10. Excudebatur et venit apud J. P. Migne, Editorem, 1865.

12. Babelon, Jean. *Peintres D'Espagne.* Paris: Les Editions Universelles,140, Boulevard Saint-Germain, 1946.

13. Baker, Charles. *The Education of the Senses.* London: Central Society of Education. Printed for Taylor and Walton, Booksellers and Publishers to the Society, Upper Gower Street, 1837.

14. Barnard, Henry. *A Tribute to Gallaudet.* Hartford: Brockell and Hutchinson, 1852.

15. Barrows, Charles M. *Transformation, The Deaf Taught to Hear.* New York: no publisher given, 1908.

16. Becker, Ulrich Thieme. *Allgemeinen Lexikon Der Bildenden Küenstler.* Leipzig: B. A. Beeman, 1915.

17. Bede, The Venerable. *Ecclesiastical History of England also the Anglo-Saxon Chronicle.* Edited by J. A. Gile. London: George Bell and Sons. 1900.

18. Bélanger, Adolphe, Professeur à l'Institution Nationale des Sourds-Muets de Paris. *Étude Bibliographique et Iconographique sur l'Abbé de l'Épée.* Paris: Librairie Paul Ritti, 21, rue de Vaugirard, 1886.

19. Bell, Alexander Melville. [a]*English Visible Speech in Twelve Lessons.* Washington, D.C.: The Volta Review, 1895.
    [b] *Sounds and Their Relations.* Salem: J. H. Coate and Co., 1881.

20. Best, Harry. *The Deaf, Their Position in Society and the Provision for their Education in the United States.* New York: Thomas Y. Crowell, 1914.

21. Boatner, Maxine Tull. *Voice of the Deaf.* Washington, D.C.: Public Affairs Press, 1959.

22. Bonet, Juan Pablo. *Reduction de las Letras y Arte para Enseñar a Hablar Los Mudos.* En Madrid: Par Francisco Abarca de Angelo. 1620.

23. Bonifaccio, Di Giovanni. *L'Arte de Cenni, con la Quale Formandosi Favella Visible, Si Tratta Della Muta Eloquenza, che non E' Altro che un Facondio Silentio.* In Vicenza: Appresso Francesco Grossi, con licenza de Superiori. MDCXVI (1616).

24. Bonuccelli, P. Giovanni. *Il Metodo Orale al Lume delle più Moderne Acquisizione Scientifiche.* Siena: Scuola Tipografica Sordomuti, 1956. Uncopyrighted.

25. Brockhaus, F. A. *Der Grosse Brockhaus.* Sechzenti Völlig Neubearbeitate, Auflage in Zwölf Bänden. Funfter Band. Wiesbaden: 1954.

26. Brugmans, J. G. Eerste Hoofdonderwijzer van het Instituut voor Doofstommen te Groningen. *De Eerste Eeuw van het Instituut voor Doofstommen te Groningen.* Groningen: Bij J. B. Wolters, 1896.

27. Bryan's *Dictionary of Painters and Engravers.* London: Geo. Bell and Sons, 1900.

28. Bulwer, John B. [a]*Chirologia or the Natural Language of the Hand.* London: Printed by Tho. Harper, and are to be sold by R. Whitaker, at his shop in Paul's Church-Yard, 1644.
    [b] *Chironomia,* or *The Art of Manual Rhetorique.* London: Printed by Tho. Harper, and are to be sold by Richard Whitaker, at his shop in Paul's Church-Yard, 1644.
    [c] *Philocophus,* or *The Deafe and Dumbe Man's Friend.* London: Humphrey Moseley, 1648.

29. Burger, H., Prof. at Univ. of Amsterdam. *Compendium of Diseases of the Ears, Nose, Throat, and Esophagus.* Third Edition. Haarlem: F. Bohn, Ltd., 1934.

30. Burnet, G., D.D. *Some Letters containing An Account of What Seemed Most Remarkable in Switzerland, Italy.* Written to T. H. R. B. Printed in Year 1687. The Fourth Letter.

31. Burnet, James, Lord Monboddo. *Of the Origin and Progress of Language.* Vol. I. Edinburgh: Printed for A. Kincaid and W. Creech, Edinburgh, and T. Cadell in the Strand, London. MDCCLXXIII (1773).

32. Cardan, Jerome. [a]*The Book of My Life.* De Vita Propria Liber, 1575. Translated from the Latin by Jean Stoner. New York: E. P. Dutton and Co., 1930.
    [b] Cardani, Hieronymi. *Quo Continentur Opuscula Miscellanea Ex Fragmentis et Paralipomenis.* Lugduni: Sumptibus Joannis Antonii Huguetan et Marci Antonii Ravaud, 1663.

33. Castro, Petri. [a]*Bayonatis Febris Maligna Punctularis Aphorismis Delineata.* Norimbergae: Ex officino endtererorum Iun, 1652.
    [b] Castro, Ezechiele Di. *La Commare, Colostro.* Verona: Francesco de Rosal, 1642.

34. Carton, L'Abbe. *L'Education des Sourds-Muets.* (In Miscellaea). Paris: A. Dubrande et M. Dupont, 1883.

35. Champlin, John Denison. *Cyclopedia of Painters and Painting.* New York: Chas. Scribner and Sons, Vol. 4, 1887.

36. Clarke School. *Alumni Bulletin.* Northampton: Published by the Alumni Association of Clarke School, October-December, 1955.

37. *Corporis Juris Civilis.* Tomus Secundus. Amstelaedami: Joannem Blaeu &e Lud. &e Dan. Elzevirios; Lugduni Batavorum; apud Franciscum Hackium, MDCLXIII (1663).

38. Cubberly, Elwood P. *History of Education*. Boston: Houghton Mifflin Co., 1920.

39. Cuevas, P. Fr. Julian Zarco. *Documenta para la Historia del Monasterio de San Lorenzo el Real de El Escorial*. Madrid: Imprenta Helenica, n.d.

40. Curtis, John Harmon. *An Essay on the Deaf and Dumb*. London: Longman, Rees, Erme, Brown, Green, and Longman, 1834.

41. Dalgarno, George. [a]Ars Signorum Vulgo Character Philosophica. Londoni: Excudebatur J. Hayes, 1661.
    [b] Didascopholus, or The Deaf and Dumb Man's Tutor. Oxford: Timo. Halton, 1680.

42. Degérando, Joseph Marie. *De L'Education des Sourds-Muets de Naissance*. Paris: Chez Mequiqnon L'Aîne Père, Editeur, 1827.

43. De Land, Fred. [a]*Dumb No Longer, Romance of the Telephone*. Washington City: Volta Bureau, 1908.
    [b] *The Story of Lipreading. Its Genesis and Development*. Washington, D.C.: The Volta Bureau, 1931.

44. De L'Épée, L'Abbé Charles Michel. [a]*Controversie Entre L'Abbé de l'Épée et Samuel Heinicke au sujet de la Veritable Maniere d'Instruire les Sourds-Muets*. Traduite de Latin par J. Alard, Officier d'Academie. Paris: Imprimerie G. Pelluard, 222, Rue Saint Jacques, 225, 1881.
    [b] *La Veritable Manière d'Instruire Les Sourds et Muets*. Paris: Chez Nyon l'Aîné, 1784.

45. Digby, Kenelme, [a]*The Nature of Bodies*. London: John Williams, 1665.
    [b] *Private Memoirs of Sir Kenelme Digby*. London: Saunders and Otley, 1827.
    [c] *The Life of Sir Kenelme Digby*, by one of his descendants. London: Longmans, Green and Co., 1896.

46. Doctor, Powrie Vaux. *Amos Kendall, Nineteenth Century Humanitarian*. Washington, D. C.: Gallaudet College Bulletin, Vol. 7, Bulletin No. 1, October, 1957.

47. Dorchain, Auguste. *Anthologie de Ronsard et de son École*. Paris: Libraire Delagrave, 1929.

48. Eby, Frederick. *The Development of Modern Education*. New York: Prentice-Hall, 1952.

49. Eby, Frederick and Arrowood, Charles Flinn. *The History and Philosophy of Education, Ancient and Medieval*. New York: Prentice-Hall, 1940.

50. Edinburgh: *A Graphic and Historical Description of the City of Edinburgh*. Vol. 1. London: Published by J. and H. S. Stoner, Chapel Street, Pentonville, 1818.

51. Elliott, Richard, Headmaster of the Asylum for the Deaf and Dumb. [a]*Lessons in Elementary Language for the Deaf and Elementary Lessons in Arithmetic*. Margate: Published by the Committee. Printed at "Keble's Gazette" Office, 1897.

^b *A Series of Lessons in Articulation and Lip-Reading.* Published by the Committee, 1897.

^c *A Series of Questions on Common Subjects.* Intended as a help to the Acquirement of Familiar and Colloquial Language by the Deaf. Margate: Printed at "Keble's Gazette" Office, 1905.

^d *A Vocabulary of Words in Common Use Arranged in the Order of Difficulty, in Six Courses.* Intended for the Elementary Instruction of the Deaf and Dumb in Language. London, Old Kent Road, and Margate: Published by the Committee at their office, 93, Cannon Street, E. C., 1878.

52. Elstad, Leonard M. ^a*Communication Problems of the Deaf*—The Gallaudet College Approach. Kendall Green, Washington, D.C.: Gallaudet College, Vol. 5, Bulletin No. 1, March 1956.

^b "The Physically Handicapped and Health Problems." *Special Education for the Exceptional,* edited by Merle E. Frampton and Elena D. Gall. Boston: Porter Sargent, Publisher, 1956.

53. Eschke, Ernst Adolf. *Lesebuch für Taubstumme.* Zweite geänderte. Linienstrasse, Nr. 110, 1805.

54. Ewing, Irene R. and Ewing, Alex W.G. ^a*Opportunity and the Deaf Child.* London: University of London Press, 1947.

^b *Speech and the Deaf Child.* Washington, D.C.: The Volta Bureau, n.d.

55. Fay, Edgar Allen, Editor. *Histories of the American Schools for the Deaf.* Washington, D.C., Volta Bureau, 1893.

56. Friedenwald, Harry. *The Jews and Medicine Essays.* Baltimore: Johns Hopkins Hospital Press, 1944.

57. Gallaudet, Edward Miner. *Life of Thomas Hopkins Gallaudet.* New York: Henry Holt and Company, 1888.

58. Glasgow: *A Brief Historical Sketch of the Origin and Progress of the Glasgow Deaf and Dumb Institution.* Glasgow: Printed for the Institution at the Scottish Guardian Office and Published by John Smith and Son, Booksellers, No. 70, St. Vincent Street, MDCCCXXXV (1835).

59. Goldstein, Max A. ^a*The Acoustic Method.* St. Louis: The Laryngoscope Press, 1939.

^b *Problems of the Deaf.* St. Louis: The Laryngoscope Press, 1933.

60. Gordon, Joseph Claybaugh. *Notes and Observations upon the Education of the Deaf.* Washington, D.C.: The Volta Bureau, 1892.

61. Gould, John. *Biographical Dictionary of Eminent Artists, Comprising Painters, Sculptors, Engravers, and Architects, from the Earliest Ages to the Present Time.* New Edition, Vol. II. London: Effingham Wilson, Royal Exchange, 1835.

62. Graser, Johann Baptist. *Samuel Heinicke, Beobachtung über Stumme.* No Publisher nor date given.

63. Gray, Forbes. *An Edinburgh Miscellany.* Edinburgh: Robert Grant and Son, 126 Princes Street, n.d.

64. Green, Francis, *Vox Oculis Subjecta.* By a Parent. London: Benjamin White, 1783.

65. Greene, D. *Manual of Articulation Teaching.* New York: Published by the Institution for the Improved Education of Deaf Mutes, 1891.

66. Groningen: *Bericht Aangaande Het Instituut tot Onderwijzing van Doven en Stommen binnen Groningen.* Groningen: J. Bolt, J. Oomkens, en J. Dikema, Boekverkopers, 1792.

67. Hardy, William G. *Children with Impaired Hearing, an Audiological Perspective.* Washington, D.C.: Government Printing Office, 1952.

68. Hartman, Arthur. *Deaf-Mutism and the Education of Deaf-Mutes by Lipreading and Articulation.* Translated and enlarged by James Patterson Cassells. London: Bailliere, Tindall and Cox, 1881.

69. Hassenpflug-Hansel. *Allgemeine Deutsche Biographie.* Erster Band. Leipzig: Verlag von Dunder und Humbolt, 1880.

70. Hatton, Joseph. *Deaf-&-Dumb Land.* London: Printed by Waterflow Brothers and Lawton, Ltd. for the Asylum for the Deaf and Dumb, Old Kent Road and Margate, n.d.

71. Heinicke, Samuel. [a]*Beobachtungen über Stumme und über die Menschliche Sprache, in Briefen von Samual Heinicke.* Erster Theil. Hamburg: In der Heroldschen Buch-handlung, 1778.
    [b] Controversie—(see 44a).
    [c] *Festgabe: Zur Samuel Heinicke Jubiläiumstagung des Bunde Deutscher Taubstummenlehrer.* Hamburg: 1927.

72. Hervas y Panduro, Lorenzo. *Escuela Española de Sordo-Mudos o Arte para Enseñarles a Escribir y Hablar el Idioma Español.* Madrid: En La Imprenta Real, Año de 1795.

73. Hill, Moritz, Inspector der Taubstummen-Anstalt zu Weissenfels.
    [a] *Beleuchtung der in dem Preussischen Gesetzen anhaltenen singülaren Bestimmungen in Betreft Taubstummer Personen nebst darauf bezuglichen Verbesserung-Vorschlägen.* Leipzig: Verlag von Carl Merseburger, 1861.
    [b] *Elementar-Lese-und Sprachbuch.* Erste Auflage, Weissenfels, September 21, 1851. Angeschlossen an die Bildersammlung, Zweite Auflage, 1858. Leipzig: Verlag von Carl Merseburger, 1870.
    [c] *Elementar-Lese-und Sprachbuch für Taubstumme.* Neubearbeitet von Fr. Krobrick, Direktor der Prov-Taubstummen-Anstalt zu Halle. Erstes Bändchen, 2-4 Schul jahr, Siebente Auflage, Preis ungebunden 80 pf. Leipzig: Verlag von Carl Merseburger, 1897.
    [d] *Die Neusten Vorschläge zur Forderung des Taubstummen-Bildungs-Wesens.* Weimar: Herman, Bohlau, 1872.

74. Hirsch, David, Lid van het bestuur en Directeur-Hoofdonder-wijzer der Inrichting voor Doofstommen-onderwijs te Rotter-dam. *Wenken, Bij de opvoeding van doofstommen voor Onders, Plee gauders en Leermeesters.* Rotterdam: Gedrukt bij J. de Jong, 1875.

75. Hodgson, Kenneth W. *The Deaf and Their Problems.* New York: Philosophical Library, 1954.

76. Hökold, Moritz. *Abbé de l'Épée und Heinicke.* Dresden: Drucke von B. C. Taubner, 1874.

77. Holder, William. *Elements of Speech.* London: Printed by T. N. for J. Martyn, Printer of The Royal Society, 1669.

78. Huisman, A., Onderwijzer aan "Effatha." *Amman, John Conrad, de grondlegger der Spreekmethode bij het onderwijs aan doofstommen.* Housden: A. Gezelle Meerburg, 1910.

79. Jäger, Victor. *Über die Behandlung welche Blinden und Taub-stummen Kindern zu Theilwerden sollte.* Stuttgart: n.p., 1830.

80. Johnson, Samuel. *A Journey to the Western Islands of Scotland.* London: W. Strahan and T. Cadell, 1775.

81. Journiac, Saint-Meard, Francois de. *Memoirs sur Les Journées de 1792, September; Mme. La Marquise Sausse-Lendry; Sicard, Roche Ambroise Cucurron; et M. Gabriel-Ami Jourdan.* Notes par M. F. S. Barriere. Paris: Firmin Didot Frères, Fils et Cie, Rue Jacob, 56, 1858.

82. Kerger, Wilhelm. *Brief an D. Michael Ernst Ettmüller.* Aus dem Lateinischen übersezt. Liebniz: den 5, April, 1704.

83. Kinniburgh, Robert. *Plates for the Deaf and Dumb as used in the Edinburgh Institute.* Edinburgh: Printed by J. Ritchie; Pub-lished by Wm. Oliphant, 22, South Bridge; and sold by M. Ogle, Glasgow, and Ogle, Duncan and Co., London, 1820.

84. Kutner, S. *A Classified Picture Vocabulary for Deaf Children.* London: George Philip and Son, n.d.

85. Lang, Robert. *Dr. John Conrad Amman, A Sketch of his Life.* Prepared for the Centenary publication of the city of Schoff-hausen and entitled Schauser, Gelerhte, und Staatsmänner. Schoffhausen: 1901.

86. Lana-Terzi, J. P. Francesco. *Prodromo.* Brescia: Par li Rizzardi, Con Licenza de' Superiori, M.DC.LXX (1670).

87. Lasso, El Lic. Io Lasso. *Tratado legal sobre los mudos.* (Copied from original manuscript in 1899, with an English translation.)

88. Laveaux, Marty. *Ouevres Francoises de Joachim du Bellay.* Paris: Alphonse Lemerre, Editeur. Tom Premiere. 1866.

89. Legre, Ludovic. *Des Memoirs de Felix et de Thomas Platter.* Traduit de l'Allemand par M. Kieffer. Marseille: H. Aubertin et G. Rolle, Libraires-Editeurs, 1900.

90. Leonardo da Vinci, *The Notebooks of.* Arranged, Rendered into English, and Introduced by Edward McCurdy. New York: George Brazmiller, 1958. First published by Reynal and Hitch-

cock, Inc., 1939.
91. Le Pere, Ch. *Statue de L'Abbé de l'Épée*, Ouevre de M. Felix Martin. Compte-Rendu de la Seance D'Inauguration présideé le 14 Mai 1879. Paris: Boucquin, Imprimeur de l'Institution Nationale des Sourds-Muets de Paris, Rue de la Sainte-Chapelle, 5, 1879.
92. Mackenzie, Catherine. *Alexander Graham Bell*, The Man Who Contracted Space. New York: Houghton Mifflin Co., 1928.
93. Mann, Edwin John. *The Deaf and Dumb*. Boston: D. K. Hitchcock, 1836.
94. Mather, Increase. *Remarkable Providences Illustrative of the Earlier Days of American Colonization*. London: Reeves and Turner, 1890.
95. McCormick, Patrick J. *History of Education*. Washington, D. C.: The Catholic Press, 1946.
96. *The Mishnah*. Translated from the Hebrew by Herbert Danby. London: Oxford University Press, 1933.
97. Morley, Henry. *The Life of Girolamo Cardano of Milan*. London: Chapman and Hall, 193, Piccadilly, MDCCCLIV (1854).
98. Müller, Fr. *Die Künstler Alter Zeiten und Volker*. Stuttgart: Verlag von Ebner und Seubert, Dritter Band, 1864.
99. Murphy, Arthur. *The Life of David Garrick, Esq*. London: Printed for J. Wright, Piccadilly, by J. F. Fort, Red Lion Passage, Fleet St., 1801.
100. Mygind, Holger, M.D. *Deaf-Mutism*. London: F. G. Rebman, 11, Adam Street, Strand, 1894.
101. Nagler, G. K. *Neues Allgemeines Künstler-Lexikon*, Bd. Sechste Lieferung. München: Verlag von Ernst August Fleischmann, 1841.
102. Peet, Harvey Prindle. *Elementary Lessons, Being a Course of Instruction for Deaf and Dumb*. New York: Baker, Pratt, and Co., 1882.
103. Peet, Isaac Lewis. *Language Lessons Destined to Introduce Young Learners, Deaf-Mutes, and Foreigners to a Correct Understanding and Use of the English Language on the Principle of Object Teaching*. New York: Baker, Pratt, and Co., 1875.
104. Petschke, August Friedrich, Lehrer der Taubstummen, Leipzig. *Allgemein Fasslicher Unterricht in der Declination de Deutschen Nenn-und Beiwörter*. Leipzig: In der Commerschen Buchhandlung, 1807.
105. Plateri, Felicis. ªDe Corporis Humani Structura et Usu, Medici Antecessoris*. Ex officina Libri III, n.d.
   ᵇ *In Hominis Affectibus Plerisque, Corpori et Animo*. Functionum Laesone, Dolore, alia ve Molestia et Vitio Incommodantibus. Basileae: Typis Conradi Waldkirchii, Libri Tres, 1614.
   ᶜ *Seu de Cognoscendis, Predicendis, Pracaundis, Curandisque Affectibus Hominis*. Basileae: Typis Conradi Waldkirchii, 1609.

d *Des Memoires de Felix et de Thomas Platter.* Traduit de l'Allemand par M. Kieffer. Marseille: H. Aubertin et G. Rolle Libraires Editeur, 1900.

106. Plato, *The Cratylus, Phaedo, Parmenides, and Timaeus of Plato.* Translated from the Greek by Thomas Taylor. London: Printed for Benjamin and John White, M.DCCC.XCIII (1793)

107. Raphel, M. Georg. *Kunst Taube und Stumme reden zu lehren.* Leipzig: A. F. Petschke; in der Sommerschen Buchhandlung, 1801.

108. Reuschert, E. *Friedrich Moritz Hill,* der Reformator des deutschen Taubtummenunterrichts; Ein Gedenkblatt zu seinem hundertjährigen Gebiertstage, mit Beiträgen hervorragender Zeitgenossen Hill's Bearbeitet. Berlin: N. 37, Selbstverlag, Templiner Strasse No. 113, 1905.

109. Ronsard, Pierre de. *Oeuvres Complet.* Nouvelle edition Publies sur les textes des les plus anciens, avec les variantes et des notes par Prosper Blanchemain. Paris: Chez P. Jannet, Libraire, 1857.

110. Rossellio, R. P. F. Cosma. *Thesaurus.* Venetius: Apud Antonium Paduanium, Bibliopolam Florentinum, MDLXXIX (1579).

111. Saulnier, V. L. *Du Bellay, L'Homme et L'Oeuvres.* Paris: Brown et Cie, 1951.

112. Schenckio, Jo. *Observationes Medicae de Capit Humano.* Basileae: Ex Officina Frobenian, 1584.

113. Schumann, Georg und Paul. *Samuel Heinickes Gesammelte Schriften.* Leipzig: Ernst Wiegandt, Verlagsbuchhandlung. (Verlagsabteilung Der Buchhandlung Alfred Lorentz), 1912.

114. Schumann, Paul. a*Samuel Heinickes Sendung.* Leipzig: Karl Sigismund, Strasse 2, 1927.
   b *Samuel Heinicke's Schriften die Taubstummenbildung.* Erste Abteilung. Leipzig: n.d.

115. Schunhoff, Hugo F. *The Teaching of Speech and by Speech in Public Residential Schools for the Deaf in the United States, 1815-1955.* Romney, West Virginia: West Virginia Schools for the Deaf and the Blind, 1957.

116. Seagle, William. *Men of Law.* From Hammurabi to Holmes. New York: Macmillan Co., 1947.

117. Seguin, Eduardo. *Educación de Los Sordomudos, Jacobo Roderiquez Pereira.* Madrid: Francisco Beltran, 1939.

118. Seiss, Joseph A. *The Children of Silence.* Philadelphia: Porter and Coates, 1887.

119. Sibscota, George. *The Deaf and Dumb Man's Discourse.* London: Printed by H. Bruges, for William Crook at the Green Dragon, without Temple-Bar, 1670.

120. Sicard, Roche Ambroise Cucurron. a*Cours D'Instruction d'un Sourd-Muet de Naissance,* Pour Servir a L'Education Des

Sourds-Muets. Paris: Chez Le Clere Libraire, Quai des Augustins, No. 39, au coin de la rue Pavée, An VII (1800).

b *Théorie des Signes.* Paris. De L'Imprimerie d'a clo, Treuttel et Wurtz, 1818.

121. Skinner, Robert T. *A Notable Family of Scots Printers.* Edinburgh: Printed privately by T. and A. Constable, Lmtd., 1927.

122. Sluizer, M. *Dr. J. C. Amman.* Amsterdam: 1934.

123. Spooner, S. *A Biographical History of Fine Arts.* New York: J. W. Bouton, 1865.

124. Streng, Alice, et al. *Hearing Therapy for Children.* New York: Grune and Stratton, 1955.

125. Syle, Henry Winter. *A Retrospect of the Education of the Deaf.* Philadelphia: Wm. R. Cullingworth, 1886.

126. *Talmud.* The New Edition of the Babylonian Talmud. Original text edited and translated into English by Michael L. Rodkinson. Boston: New Talmud Publishing Co., 1903.

127. Tomas, T. Navarro. *Juan Pablo Bonet.* Barcelona: Imprenta de la Casa de Curitat, 1920.

128. Tarra, M. l'Abbé Jules, Directeur et Professeur à l'École des Pauvres. *Esquisse Historique et Court Exposé de la Methode Suivie pour l'Instruction des Sourds-Muets de la Paroisse et du Diocèse de Milan.* Traduction de M. M. A. Dubranle and M. Dupont, Professeurs à l'Institution Nationale des Sourds-Muets de Paris. Paris: Libraire ch: Delgrave, 15 Rue Soufflot, 1883.

129. Uchermann, V. *Les Sourds-Muets En Norvége.* Publié par les Soins de l'État. Traduit du Norvegien par Joachim Nicolaysen et Théophile Chauvin. Christiania: Abb. Cammermeyer, Editeur, 1901.

130. Ulster: *Some Information Respecting the Origin, Constitution, Object, and Operations of the Ulster Society for Promoting the Education of the Deaf and Dumb, and the Blind, Especially Designed for the Use of the Societies Auxiliaries.* Belfast: Printed for the Society, MDCCCXLVI (1846).

131. Van Helmont, F. M. B. *Alphabeti, vere Naturalis Hebraici Brevissima Delineatio.* Sulzbaci: Typis Abrahamis Lichenthaleri, Anno M.DC.LVII (1657).
Part II—Pictures
Anno M.DC.LXVII (1667).

132. Van Praagh, William. *Lessons for the Instruction of Deaf and Dumb Children in Speaking, Lipreading, Reading, and Writing.* London: Trubner and Co., Ludgate Hill, 1884. Price 2s. 6d.

133. Wallis, Johannes. *De Loquella Sive Sonorum Foratione Tractatus Grammatico-Physicus.* Editio Sexta. Lugduni, Batavorum: Apud Jo. Arn. Langerak, 1727.

134. Walther, Eduard. *Die Königliche Taubstummenanstalt zu Berlin.* Berlin: von Elwin Staude, 1888.

135. Waring, E. S. *The Deaf in the Past and Present Time.* Grinnell, Iowa: E. S. Waring, Job Printer, 1896.
136. Watson, Joseph. [a]*Instruction of the Deaf and Dumb.* London: Printed and sold by Darton and Harvey, Grace-church Street; To be had also of the author at the Asylum, Kent Road, 1809.
   [b] *Plates Illustrative of the Vocabulary for the Deaf and Dumb.* London: Harvey and Company, 1810.
137. Willman, Otto. *Lexikon der pädagogik Im Verein mit Fachmännern und unter Besonderer Mitwirkung.* Zweiter Band. Freiburg im Breisgau: Ernst M. Roloff, 1913.
138. Yale, Caroline A. *Years of Building.* The Dial Press, New York. MCMXXXI (1931).

ARTICLES

139. Baker, Charles. "Papers on Deaf-Mute Education." *Quarterly Journal of Education.* No. XIV. (April 1834). Privately reprinted, 1862.
140. "The Braidwood Family." *American Annals of the Deaf and Dumb.* Vol. XXII. (1878).
141. *Clinical Excerpts.* Vol. 23 (1957).
142. The Columbia Encyclopedia. "Agricola, Rudolphus." 2nd edition. (1950).
143. *Cleveland Plain Dealer.* June 12, 1955.
144. Doyle, Thomas S. "The Virginia Institution for the Education of the Deaf and Dumb." *Histories of American Schools for the Deaf and Dumb and Blind.* Vol. I. (1893).
145. *Edinburgh Evening News.* September 30, 1936.
146. Elstad, Leonard M. "Historical Backgrounds of Types of Schools and Methods of Communication." *American Annals of the Deaf.* Vol. 103, March, 1958.
147. Encyclopedia Britannica. [a]"Babylonian Law." Vol. III, 11th edition.
   [b] "Galen." Vol. XIX, 11th edition.
   [c] "Justinian I." Vol. XV, 11th edition.
   [d] "Medicine." Vol. XVIII, 11th edition.
   [e] "Pliny, the Elder." Vol. XXI, 11th edition.
148. Fauth, Betty LaVerne and Warren Wesley. "A Study of the Proceedings of Conventions of American Instructors of the Deaf, from 1850 to 1949." *American Annals of the Deaf,* March, 1950.
149. Fortune, George J. "A Pattern of Living for Deaf Children and Their Parents." *Oralism and Auralism.* Transactions of the 31st Annual Meeting of National Forum on Deafness and Speech Pathology. February, 1949.
150. Franke, Karl. "The Deaf in Post-War Germany." *The Volta Review,* June, 1948.

151. Gallaudet, Edward Miner. "Results of Articulation Teaching at Northampton." *American Annals of the Deaf and Dumb*. Vol. XIX. 1874.

152. Greenberger, D. "Hill's Method: Moritz Hill." *American Annals of the Deaf and Dumb*. Vol. XIX. (1874).

153. Grosvenor, Elsie May Bell. [a]"My Father." *The Volta Review*. (March, 1950).
     [b] "My Father, Alexander Graham Bell." *The Volta Review*. (August, 1951).

154. Grosvenor, Lillian. "Deaf Children Learn to Talk at Clarke School." *The National Geographic*. Vol. CVII, No. 3, March, 1955.

155. Holder, William. [a]*Philosophical Transactions*. Vol. II. London: In the Savoy, Printed by T. N. for John Martyn at the Bell, a little without Temple-Bar. (1669).
     [b] "Some Reflections on Dr. Wallis, his letters there inserted." *Supplement to the Philosophical Transactions*. (1678).

156. Iowa School for the Deaf. "This is Your Life, Mr. Bell." *Volta Review*. Vol. 57, No. 8 (October, 1955).

157. *The Jewish Encyclopedia*. "Deaf and Dumb in Jewish Law." New York: Funk and Wagnalls Co., Vol. IV.

158. Jones, Henry, *Philosophical Transactions* (From Year 1700 to year 1720). Vol. V. The Second Edition. London: Printed J. and J. Knapton, et al., 1731.

159. Kuder, K. "The Hard of Hearing in Post-War Germany." *The Volta Review*, June, 1948.

160. Lane, Helen S. Report on studies by Heider and Heider at Clarke School. *American Annals of the Deaf*. Vol. 90, No. 4.

161. Lowthorp, John. "The Philological and Miscellaneous Papers." Published and Dispersed in *The Philosophical Transactions and Collections*. Abridged and Dispersed under General Heads. Vol. III in Two Parts. The Fourth Edition. London: Printed by T. W. for J. and J. Knapton, D. Midwinter, and A. Ward, A. Bettsworth, et. al. MDCCXXXI (1731).

162. McClure, William J. "The Controversy over Methods." *The Silent Worker*. (October, 1954).

163. "On the Oral Education of the Deaf and Dumb." A paper read at the Teachers' Conference, January 10, 1878. Reprinted from Journal of Education. London: 11, Fitzroy Square W.

164. Peet, Harvey Prindle. "Memoirs on Origin and Early History of the Art of Instructing the Deaf and Dumb." *American Annals of the Deaf and Dumb*. Vol. III, No. III, (April, 1851).

165. *Penny Cyclopedia*. [a]"Biographical Notices." Vol. IV., n.d.
     [b] "On the Education of the Deaf and Dumb." Vol. VII, (1857).

166. Porter, Samuel. "Bibliography." *American Annals of the Deaf and Dumb*. Vol. I. 1848.

167. *The Quarterly Review of Deaf-Mute Education.* Edited and issued under the direction of the following committee: E. W. Dawson, H. N. Dixon, R. Elliott, J. Howard, S. Schontheil, W. Sleight, W. Stainer, W. Van Praagh. Vol. IV. 1895, 1896, 1897. London: Published at the Office, Stainer House, Paddington Green, W., 1898.

168. Rae, Luzerne. ^aL'Abbé de l'Épée, from Bebiàn's "Eloge Historique de Charles Michel de l'Épée." *American Annals of the Deaf and Dumb.* Vol. I. (January, 1848).
   [b] "The Great Peril of Sicard." *American Annals of the Deaf and Dumb.* Vol. I. (January, 1848).
   [c] "Historical Sketch of Instruction of Deaf and Dumb before de l'Épée." *American Annals of Deaf and Dumb.* Vol. I. No. IV. (July, 1848).
   [d] "A Monument to Heinicke." *American Annals of the Deaf and Dumb.* Vol. I. No. III (April, 1848).

169. Rau, Natalie. "Work for the Deaf in Russia." *The Volta Review,* January, 1948.

170. Rew, Ada. "Deaf Schools in Japan." *The Audiogram.* Vol. XXXI, No. 1, San Diego Hearing Society, January-February, 1957.

171. Saegert, C. W. "Education of Deaf and Dumb in Prussia." Translated from the German by Benjamin Talbot. *American Annals of the Deaf and Dumb.* Vol. IX, No. IX. (October, 1857).

172. Sanders, Jennings B. "Gallaudet College." *Higher Education.* September, 1954.

173. Schumann, Paul. "The Place of the Deaf in the New Reich." Translated by Tobias Brill. *American Annals of the Deaf.* Vol. LXXIX, No. 3, May, 1934.

174. *Magazine for the Scottish Deaf.* Edinburgh: October-November, 1929.

175. *The Scots Magazine.* Edinburgh: Printed by W. Sands, A. Murray, and J. Cochran: ^aMDCCLXVI. Vol. XXXI. (January, 1766).
   [b] MDCCLXVII. (August, 1767).
   [c] MDCCLXIX. (July 15, 1769).

176. *The Scotsman.* Edinburgh: April 2, 1929; October 1, 1936; July 23, 1937; November 12, 1952; November 14, 1952.

177. Snowden, W. H. "Les Sourd-Muets de 1851." *The Volta Review.* Vol. 53. (December, 1953).

178. Stovel, Laura. "Alexander Graham Bell in the Hall of Fame." *The Volta Review.* (August, 1951).

179. Streng, Alice. "On Improving the Teaching of Language." *American Annals of the Deaf.* Vol. 103, No. 5, Nov. 1958.

180. Taylor, Wallace W. and Isabella. "The Education of Physically Handicapped Children in Austria." *Exceptional Children.* Vol. 25, No. 9, May, 1959.

181. Taylor, Wallace W. and Isabella. "The Education of Physically

Handicapped Children in France." *Exceptional Children.* Vol. 26, No. 2, October, 1959.

182. Taylor, Wallace W. and Isabella. "The Education of Physically Handicapped Children in Portugal." *Exceptional Children.* Vol. 26, No. 1, September, 1959.

183. Taylor, Wallace W. and Isabella. "The Education of Physically Handicapped Children in Yugoslavia." *Exceptional Children.* Vol. 26, No. 3, November, 1959.

184. Thornton, William. "Cadmus: Essay on Teaching of Deaf or Surd and Consequently Dumb to Speak." *Transactions of the American Philosophical Society.* Vol. III. (1893).

185. Utley, Jean. "The Preschool Deaf Child." *The Palmetto Leaf.* South Carolina School for the Deaf and Blind, Cedar Springs, South Carolina. Vol. XLIV, No. 4 and No. 5, November, 1942.

186. Van Uden, A. "Observations on the Education of the Deaf in the Netherlands and the U.S.A." *The Volta Review.* Vol. 62, No. 1, January, 1960.

187. Wallis, John. [a]"A Defense of the Royal Society, In Answer to the Cavils of Dr. Holder." *Supplement to the Philosophical Transactions.* (1678).
[b] "Letter of Wallis to Boyle." *Philosophical Transactions.* (1670).

188. *Weekly Scotsman.* Edinburgh: January 1, 1938; January 15, 1938.

PUBLIC DOCUMENTS

189. *British Museum General Catalogue of Printed Books.* London: William Clowes and Sons. Vol. II. 1931.

REPORTS

190. Report of the Committee of the Connecticut Asylum for the Education and Instruction of Deaf and Dumb Persons. Hartford: Hartford-Hudson and Co.
[a] First Annual Report. 1817.
[b] Second Annual Report. 1818.
[c] Third Annual Report. 1819.

191. Report of the Edinburgh Institution for the Deaf and Dumb. Established June 25, 1810. Edinburgh: Printed at the Institution, 1841.

192. Report of the Proceedings of the International Congress on the Education of the Deaf, held at Milan, September 6th to 11th. Taken from the English Official Minutes, read by A. A. Kinsey. London: W. H. Allen and Co., 1880.

193. Report of the Proceedings of the World's Congress of Instructors of the Deaf and the 13th Convention of the American In-

structors of the Deaf. Washington, D.C.: Supplement to American Annals of the Deaf, 1893.

194. Report of the Proceedings of the American Association to Promote the Teaching of Speech to the Deaf. 4th Summer Meeting. Chautauqua, New York, July, 1894.

195. Report of the Proceedings of the World's Congress of the Deaf and the Report of the 7th Convention of the National Association for the Deaf, St. Louis, Missouri, 1904.

196. Report of the Proceedings of the International Conference on the Education of the Deaf. Edinburgh: The Darien Press, 1907.

197. Report of the Proceedings of the International Congress for the Education of the Deaf. West Trenton, New Jersey: New Jersey School for the Deaf, 1933.

198. Report of the Proceedings of the International Congress for the Care of the Deaf-Mute. Groningen: 1950.

199. Report of the Proceedings of the Second World Congress of the Deaf. Zagreb, Yugoslavia: Univergum, 1955.

200. Report of the Proceedings of the 37th Meeting of the Convention of American Instructors of the Deaf. Washington, D. C.: U.S. Gov. Printing Office, 1956.

201. Report of the Proceedings of the Congress for the Educational Treatment of Deafness. Manchester: Manchester Univ. Press, 1958.

202. Der Prospekt des Leipziger Institute von Jahre 1778.

203. Stevenson, Elwood A. "Report of the Conference on Nomenclature." *American Annals of the Deaf.* Vol. 83. No. I. (January, 1938).

APPENDIX TO THE BIBLIOGRAPHY

CHAPTER 10 REFERENCES

A1. Babbidge, H. S. *Education of the Deaf.* A report to the Secretary of Health, Education and Welfare by his Advisory Committee on the Education of the Deaf. Washington, D.C.: U.S. Government Printing Office, 0-765-119, 1965.

A2. Beebe, H. H. *A guide to help the severely hard-of-hearing child.* Basel, Switzerland: S. Karger, 1953.

A3. Bellugi, U. and Studdert-Kennedy, M. (Eds.). *Signed and spoken language, Dahlem Workshop Report-Berlin.* Deerfield Beach, Florida: Verlag Chemie International, 1980.

A4. Bergstrom, L. Congenital deafness. In J. L. Northern (Ed.). *Hearing disorders.* Boston: Little, Brown, 1976.

A5. Blackwell, P. M. *Sentences and other systems.* Washington, D. C.: A. G. Bell Association for the Deaf, 1978.

A6. Bradford, L. J. (Ed.). *Physiological measure of the audio-vestibular system*. New York: Academic Press, 1975.

A7. Calvert, D. R. The rubella epidemic of 1964: problems and response. *Journal of the American Optometric Association,* 1969, 40, 1-5.

A8. Calvert, D. R. and Silverman, S. R. *Speech and deafness: a text for learning and teaching*. Washington, D. C.: A. G. Bell Association for the Deaf, 1975.

A9. "Colorado Conference." *Education of the Deaf, the challenge and the charge: a report of the National Conference on education of the deaf.* Colorado Springs, April, 1967. Washington, D. C.: Superintendent of Documents, U.S. Government Printing Office, 1967.

A10. Craig, W. N. and Barkuloo, H. W. (Eds.). *Psychologists to deaf chilren: a developing perspective*. Pittsburgh: University of Pittsburgh, 1968.

A11. Davis, H. (Ed.). The young deaf child: Identification and management. *Acta Oto-laryngologica.* Sup. 206, 1965.

A12. Doctor, P.V. (Ed.). *Report of the Proceedings of the International Congress on Education of the Deaf and the 41st meeting of the Convention of American Instructors of the Deaf*. Washington, D.C.: U.S. Government Printing Office, 1964.

A13. Eagles, E. (Ed.). *Human communication and its disorders*. Vol. 3 of D. B. Tower, (Editor-in-Chief). *The nervous system*. Commemorating the 25th Anniversary of the National Institute of Neurological and Communicative Disorders and Stroke. New York: Raven Press, 1975.

A14. Elliot, L. L. (Ed.). *Psychology and the handicapped child*. DHEW Publication No. OE773-05000. Washington, D. C.: Office of Education, U.S. Department of Health, Education and Welfare, U.S. Government Printing Office, 1974.

A15. Elliot, L. Research on the language acquisition of hearing impaired children. In S. K. Hirsh, D. H. Eldredge, I. J. Hirsh, and S. R. Silverman, (Eds.). *Hearing and Davis.* St. Louis: Washington University Press, 1976.

A16. Elliott, L. L. and Armbruster, V.A. Possible effects of the delay of early treatment of deafness. *Journal of Speech and Hearing Research,* 1967, *10*(2), 209-224.

A17. Feinmesser, M. and Tell, I. Evaluation of methods for detecting hearing impairment in infancy and early childhood. *Maternal and Child Health Service*, Report No. 06-480-2, U.S. Department of Health, Education and Welfare, 1975. (Abstracted in *Archives of Otolaryngology,* 1976, *102*, 297-299.

A18. Fraser, G. *The causes of profound deafness in childhood*. Baltimore: Johns Hopkins University Press, 1976.

A19. Furth, H. G. *Thinking without language: psychological implications of deafness* New York: The Free Press, 1966.

A20. Garretson, M.D. Total Communication. In R. Frisina (Ed.). *A bicentennial monograph on hearing impairment: trends in the U.S.A.* Washington, D. C.: A. G. Bell Association for the Deaf, 1976.

A21. Gentile, A. and McCarthy, B. *Additional handicapping conditions among hearing-impaired students, United States: 1971-72.* Washington, D. C.: Office of Demographic Studies, Gallaudet College, Series D, No. 14, 1973.

A22. Griffiths, C. (Ed.) *International conference on auditory techniques.* Springfield, Illinois: Charles C Thomas, 1974.

A23. Jensema, C. and Fitzgerald, M. Background and initial audience characteristics of the closed-caption television system. *American Annals of the Deaf,* 1981, *126*(1), 32-36.

A24. Konigsmark, B. S. and Gorlin, R. J. *Genetic and metabolic deafness.* Philadelphia: W. B. Saunders, 1976.

A25. Kretschmer, R. and Kretschmer, L. W. *Language development and intervention with the hearing impaired.* Baltimore: University Park Press, 1978.

A26. Levitt, H. and Nye, P.W. (Eds.). *Proceedings of the Conference on Sensory Training Aids for the Hearing Impaired.* Washington, D.C.: National Academy of Engineering, 1971.

A27. Ling, D. An auditory approach to the education of deaf children. *Audecibel,* 1964, *13*, 96-101.

A28. Ling, D. *Speech and the hearing impaired Child: theory and practice.* Washington, D.C.: A. G. Bell Association for the Deaf, 1975.

A29. Mayberry, R. I. Manual communication. In H. Davis and S. R. Silverman, (Eds.). *Hearing and deafness.* New York: Rinehart and Winston, 1978.

A30. Mencher, G. T. (Ed.). *Early identification of hearing loss.* New York: S. Karger, 1976.

A31. "New Orleans Conference." Stuckless, R. (Ed.). *Research on behavioral aspects of deafness.* New Orleans, May, 1965. Washington, D.C.: U.S. Department of Health Education and Welfare, Vocational Rehabilitation Administration, 1965.

A32. Perry, A. L. and Silverman, S. R. Speechreading. In H. Davis and S. R. Silverman (Eds.). *Hearing and deafness.* New York: Rinehart and Winston, 1978.

A33. Pollack, D. *Educational audiology for the limited hearing infant.* Springfield, Illinois: Charles C Thomas, 1970.

A34. Rainer, J. D., Altschuler, K. Z., Kallman, F. J., and Deming, W. E. (Eds.). *Family and mental health problems in a deaf population.* New York: New York State Psychiatric Institute, 1963.

A35. Rawlings, B., Trybus, R., and Biser, J. *A guide to college/career programs for deaf students.* Washington, D.C. and Rochester, N.Y.: Gallaudet College and National Technical Institute for the Deaf, 1981.

A36. Schein, J.D. *The deaf community*. Washington, D.C.: Gallaudet College Press, 1968.

A37. Silverman, S. R. Priorities in service delivery to the communicatively disadvantaged: rehabilitation needs. *Annals of Otology, Rhinology, and Laryngology*, 1980, Sup. 74, 89-5, 15-18.

A38. Silverman, S. R. Speech training then and now: a critical review. In I. Hochberg, H. Levitt, and M. J. Osberger, (Eds.). *Proceedings of the Conference on the Speech of the Hearing Impaired: Research, Training and Personnel Preparation*. Washington, D. C.: A. G. Bell Association for the Deaf, 1981. (In press)

A39. Simmons, F. B. Automated hearing screening test for newborns: The Crib-o-gram. In G. T. Mencher (Ed.). *Early identification of hearing loss*. New York: S. Karger, 1976.

A40. Simmons, F. B. Identification of hearing loss in infants and young children. *Otolaryngolic clinics of North America*, 1978, II: 1, 19-28.

A41. Simmons-Martin, A. The oral/aural procedure: theoretical basis and rationale. *Volta Review*, 1972, *74*, 541-551.

A42. Stark, R. E. (Ed.). *Sensory capabilities of hearing impaired children*. Baltimore: University Park Press, 1974.

A43. Stepp, R. E., Jr. (Guest Ed.). Symposium on research and utilization of educational media for teaching the deaf-back to media: how to use better what you already have. *American Annals of the Deaf*, 1980, *125*(6), 615-884.

A44. Stokoe, W. C., Casterline, D. C., and Croneberg, C. G. *A dictionary of American Sign Language on linguistic principles*. Washington, D. C.: Gallaudet College Press, 1965.

A45. Streng, A. H. *Syntax, speech and hearing: applied linguistics for teachers of children with language and hearing disabilities*. New York: Grune and Stratton, 1972.

A46. Stuckless, R. (Guest Ed.). Deafness and rubella: infants in the 60's, adults in the 80's. *American Annals of the Deaf*, 1980, *125*(8), 959-1030.

A47. Trybus, R. J., Karchmer, M. A., Kerstetter, P. P. and Hicks, W. The demographics of deafness resulting from maternal rubella. *American Annals of the Deaf*, 1980, *125*(8), 977-984.

A48. Weir, R. H. Some questions on the child's learning phonology. In F. Smith and G. H. Miller (Eds.). *The genesis of language*. Cambridge, Mass.: M.I.T. Press, 1966.

Chronology

500 B.C.	Hebrew Law	
460 B.C.	Hippocrates	
386 B.C.	Socrates	
77 A.D.	Pliny, The Elder	
170 A.D.	Galen	
530 A.D.	Justinian Code	
700 A.D.	Bede	

1450-1600

1443-1485	Agricola	(Netherlands)
1501-1576	Cardan	(Italy)
1520-1584	Ponce de Leon	(Spain)
?	Pascha	(Germany)
1522-1560	du Bellay	(France)
1524-1585	Ronsard	(France)
1526-1579	El Mudo	(Spain)
1531-1598	Schenk	(Germany)
1530-1614	Platter	(Germany)
1591	Alberti	(Germany)

1600-1700

1579-1620	Bonet	(Spain)
1615-1619 (known)	de Carrión	(Spain)
1614-1684	Bulwer	(England)
1616	Bonifacio	(Italy)
1642	di Castro	(Italy)
1655	Deusing	(Netherlands)
1665	Digby	(England)
1667	Van Helmont	(Germany)
1670	Lana-Terzi	(Italy)
1616-1698	Holder	(England)
1616-1703	Wallis	(England)
1669-1724	Amman	(Netherlands)
1670	Sibscota	(England)
1685	Burnet	(England)

1700-1800

1673-1740	Raphel	(Germany)
1698-1774	H. Baker	(England)
1712-1789	de l'Épée	(France)
1715-1780	Pereira	(France)
1715-1806	T. Braidwood	(England)
1729-1790	Heinicke	(Germany)
1735-1809	Hervas	(Spain)
1757	Ernaud	(France)
1742-1822	Sicard	(France)
1777	Arnoldi	(Germany)
1779	Deschamps	(France)
1783	Green	(United States)
1784	Silvestri	(Italy)
1753-1828	H. Guyot	(Netherlands)
1765-1829	Watson	(England)
1766-1811	Eschke	(Germany)
1766-1841	Graser	(Germany)
1772-1842	Degérando	(France)
1789-1839	Bébian	(France)
1793	Thornton	(United States)

1800-1900

1787-1851	T. Gallaudet	(United States)
1790- ?	C. Guyot	(Netherlands)
1796-1859	Pendola	(United States)
1800-1883	d'Alea	(Italy)
?	Mann	(Spain)
?	Hernandez	(Spain)
1801-1874	Valade-Gabel	(France)
1801-1876	Howe	(United States)
1803-1874	C. Baker	(England)
1810	Stafford	(United States)
? -1819	J. Braidwood	(United States)
1812	Kinniburgh	(England)
1819	Arrowsmith	(England)
1805-1874	Hill	(Germany)
1825	Jäger	(Germany)
1812-1827	Neumann	(Germany)
1813-1895	Hirsch	(Netherlands)
1816-1897	Arnold	(England)
1813-1825	T. Braidwood	(England)
1832-1889	Tarra	(Italy)
1834-1886	Balestra	(Italy)
1850-1880	Elliott	(England)
1854-1894	Alings	(Netherlands)

1856	Kendall	(United States)
1862	Hull	(United States)
1867	Rogers	(United States)
1869	Fuller	(United States)
1877	Kinsey	(England)
1878	Westervelt	(United States)
1837-1917	E. Gallaudet	(United States)
1847-1922	Bell	(United States)

Index